X

Theories and Principles of Occupational Therapy

The Authors

Mary Young trained as an occupational therapist at Dorset House School of Occupational Therapy, Oxford. She has practised in the UK, the USA and most recently, in Ireland where, until 1990, she was head of the School of Occupational Therapy at Trinity College, Dublin.

Evelyn Quinn taught psychology to occupational therapy students during the 1970s and 1980s, first at St Joseph's College of Occupational Therapy in Dublin, and later at Trinity College, Dublin. Dr Quinn currently lectures on cognitive development at University College, Dublin.

For Churchill Livingstone:

Publisher: Mary Law
Editorial Co-ordination: Editorial Resources Unit
Production Controller: Nancy Henry
Design: Design Resources Unit
Sales Promotion Executive: Hilary Brown

Theories and Principles of Occupational Therapy

Mary E. Young DipCOT MEd MA PhD

Evelyn Quinn PhD

CHURCHILL LIVINGSTONE
EDINBURGH LONDON MADRID MELBOURNE NEW YORK AND TOKYO 1992

CHURCHILL LIVINGSTONE
Medical Division of Longman Group UK Limited

Distributed in the United States of America by Churchill
Livingstone Inc., 650 Avenue of the Americas, New York,
N.Y. 10011, and by associated companies, branches and
representatives throughout the world.

First published 1992

ISBN 0-443-04060-5

British Library Cataloguing in Publication Data
A catalogue record for this book is available from the
British Library.

Library of Congress Cataloging in Publication Data
Young, Mary E., Ph. D.
    Theories and principles of occupational therapy/Mary
E. Young, Evelyn Quinn.
        p.   cm.
    Includes index.
    ISBN 0-443-04060-5
    1. Occupational therapy. I. Quinn, Evelyn.   II. Title.
    [DNLM: 1. Occupational Therapy. WB 555 Y74t]
RM737.Y68 1992
615.8'515–dc20
DNLM/DLC
for Library of Congress

Produced by Longman Singapore Publishers (Pte.) Ltd.
Printed in Singapore

Preface

In the course of their education, occupational therapy students follow a wide-ranging syllabus. Curricula, however diverse they may be, necessarily include practical subjects and a range of academic subjects whose content is largely theoretical. From an early point in professional training, students are exposed to theories pertaining to health, illness, learning, development and adjustment – all of which need to be integrated and evaluated. Qualified occupational therapists have traditionally based their practice on a broad theoretical base. While this is appropriate, in view of humankind's complexity, it can lead to professional unease. Many practitioners are unclear about the demarcation lines between the various health professions, and the very identity of occupational therapy has been called into question, or at least subjected to intense scrutiny. A core issue in this debate concerns the theories which have most relevance to the practice of occupational therapy.

In this book, we review the theories and principles that appear to be most relevant and indicate how these bear upon practice. Thus, Chapter 3 identifies and discusses influential frames of reference, and subsequent chapters deal with concepts relating to development, learning and activity. Elsewhere, we consider the general relationship between theoretical perspectives and approaches to health care (Ch. 2), and the relevance of occupational therapy to work and leisure (Ch. 8). However, our greatest emphasis is on the nature and role of activity (Chs 6 and 7) as we believe that it is the therapeutic use of activity that gives the profession its unique identity.

As, throughout the text, we use terms such as *theories, concepts, frames of reference* and *paradigms* with something approaching gay abandon, we decided at the planning stage to include a chapter which would define and discuss these terms. Obviously, the only logical place for such a chapter is at the beginning, as otherwise the terms would have to be introduced without explanation. Chapter 1 is therefore relatively difficult, in that it deals with abstract issues, including that of the nature of theories. Our discussion of this issue draws on concepts from the philosophy of science, and highlights criteria for distinguishing genuinely scientific theories from those that are not logically entitled to claim the status of science. We make the point that all theories – even those within the physical sciences – are provisional, in the sense that they can never be proved true nor established with absolute certainty. We have elaborated arguments in this area for a number of reasons. In the first place, we feel that this focus will help students to understand more fully the nature and limitations of theories. Secondly, we hope to promote insight into why competing theories prevail in any given field. (As teachers will no doubt have discovered, students tend to be puzzled by the proliferation of theories and too often want to be told which is the 'right' one.) Finally, philosophers of science have stressed the importance of a critical attitude, and we would wish our readers to be aware that to be critical is not necessarily to be negative. Criticism can be valuable and constructive, provided its basis is rational.

At a sociological level, radical changes in the field of health care are currently under way in western countries. Traditions of care, particularly institutional care, have been criticised and found wanting, and health care policies now focus on the community. Our final chapter includes a review of the issues raised by the recent change to community care and considers possible implications of this for occupational therapy.

Friends, acquaintances and professional colleagues have asked, for a number of years, 'what actually *is* occupational therapy?' Teaching students has forced us to try to find some answers which we now submit for discussion.

We fully acknowledge the work of all those we quote and offer them our grateful thanks. Our thanks are also due to the editors at Churchill Livingstone, who have shown us remarkable tolerance and who have been unfailingly supportive.

M. E. Y.
E. Q.

Contents

1. Terms and definitions

OCCUPATIONAL THERAPY: DEFINITIONS AND SCOPE

Definitions

Since occupational therapy was formally established early in the twentieth century, much progress has been made in delineating its particular objectives. As is the case for all therapeutic movements, this process has been gradual. In America, the founding country, many attempts at definition have been made over the years. Most lacked comprehensiveness, and Reed & Sanderson (1983) have identified a number of important criteria which they failed to meet. Eventually, a definition fulfilling the essential criteria was accepted by the American Occupational Therapy Association (AOTA) in 1981 (see Box 1.1)

This definition has been quoted in full because it has several merits. Firstly, its status is such that it was incorporated in American state licensure bills. Secondly, it emphasises the purposeful nature of occupational therapy, which is the special concern of this book. Thirdly, it is sufficiently comprehensive to coincide with definitions from other countries, or with less specific definitions which are, at the same time, in agreement on essentials.

Other definitions

Mocellin (1984) writes that occupational therapy is:

the health profession which teaches competent behaviour in the areas of living, learning, and working to individuals experiencing illness, developmental deficits, and/or physical and psychosocial dysfunction.

Turner's (1981) definition succinctly highlights the 'wholeness' of the human being:

Occupational therapy is the treatment of the whole person by his active participation in purposeful living.

1

Box 1.1   AOTA definition of occupational therapy

Occupational therapy is the use of purposeful activity with individuals who are limited by physical injury or illness, psychosocial dysfunction, developmental or learning disabilities, poverty and cultural differences or the aging process in order to maximise independence, prevent disability and maintain health.

The practice encompasses evaluation, treatment and consultation. Specific occupational therapy services include: teaching daily living skills; developing perceptual-motor skills and sensory integrative functioning; developing play skills and prevocational and leisure capacities; designing, fabricating or applying selected orthotic and prosthetic devices or selective adaptive equipment; using specifically designed crafts and exercises to enhance functional performance; administering and interpreting tests such as manual muscle and range of motion, and adapting environment for the handicapped. These services are provided individually, in groups, or through social systems.

A third definition, this time from Europe, is that agreed upon by Committee of Occupational Therapists for the European Communities (COTEC) members in 1989 (cited in 'Occupational Therapy' – produced monthly by the Association of Occupational Therapists of Ireland – May 1989.):

Occupational therapists assess and treat people using purposeful activity to prevent disability and develop independent function.

Taken together, these definitions highlight the role of the occupational therapist as being fundamentally a teaching one, and stress that the therapist's concern is with the whole person; thus, the approach is not a reductionist one. Similarly, they highlight the concept of purposeful activity which, although central to the practice of occupational therapy, has at times been abandoned in definitions because of its purported all-embrasive scope. However, what is needed is a concise definition which at the same time embraces the profession's scope, encompassing the ideas expressed in the lengthier AOTA definition.

While the AOTA definition has the undeniable merit of comprehensiveness, it was drawn up for legal purposes and is rather too elaborate for conventional use. Certainly, a student or practitioner, faced with the all-too-frequent question, 'What exactly is occupational therapy?' would be unlikely to reply by quoting it in full. However, the AOTA definition, as it stands, is certainly useful for academic purposes.

Practitioners

The AOTA definition makes it clear that occupational therapists serve a wide range of individuals. The knowledge required for practice must, therefore, be equally extensive. As students know all too well, dysfunction can only be appreciated in the context of normal functioning and development – at both physical and psycho-social levels. While there is still much to be learned in these areas, our knowledge continues to grow, and this growth creates its own problems.

In 1917, when the National Society for the Promotion of Occupational Therapy was set up in New York, less was known about human development than is known today. Underlying the subsequent expansion of knowledge is the fact that manpower concentration in developed countries has changed dramatically, so that more people are working in the service professions than ever before. This means that there are not only ever-increasing numbers of occupational therapists, but also more educators and researchers in academic fields which bear upon training. This 'knowledge-based' characteristic of modern society (Bell 1973) has both advantages and disadvantages for professional growth – a great deal of useful information is imparted, but much else is mere 'noise'.

The practitioners of any profession bear the burden of sifting from the total informational input, historical and contemporary, that which is relevant to their work. Happily, this information is never imparted in a vacuum, but – at least in an academic context – is organised into concepts, principles and theories. Knowledge may further be imparted by way of paradigms and models.

Concepts

Concepts are abstractions from reality. We form concepts when we classify objects, events and relationships on the basis of some quality, for example, similarity, difference or usage. Concepts develop early in life. Even a very young child will know that a knife is different from a cup on the basis of size, constituent material and usage. In other words, in knowing what the term means, the child has abstracted the common qualities of knives necessary to develop the idea or concept of 'knifeness'.

Adults (as we know from Piaget) are conceptually more sophisticated than children, and employ a variety of concepts to deal with abstract issues or issues of relationship. The terms 'energy' and 'health' are examples at this level. It should, however, be noted that possibilities for disagreement are inherent in concepts of this type: it is not unknown for people to argue late into the night about concepts pertaining to 'freedom', 'democracy' or 'the meaning of life'.

Conceptualisation at abstract levels may pose problems for researchers and practitioners. It is difficult to enquire into, or report on, concepts such as intelligence, aptitude or dysfunction, unless one specifies in advance what these terms imply. In these circumstances, meaning may be specified by operationalising the concept; that is, by defining it in terms of some clear criterion such as a test result. Intelligence as IQ, or dexterity as performance on an appropriate test are common operational definitions.

Operational definitions are typically used when it is felt necessary to define a concept with precision. An occupational therapist might, therefore, define dexterity in terms of a result on a measure such as The Crawford Small Parts Dexterity Test. This kind of approach can be useful in facilitating communication, but it does not actually add very much to our understanding of the concept, 'dexterity'. The concept is defined in terms of itself, and so is logically circular. What is essential is that some other criterion be developed to validate the test-result concept. Therapists can therefore generate their own validatory criteria with reference to, say, how skilfully the individual uses basic tools in everyday living tasks.

It is actually impossible to define concepts with any kind of ultimate precision. Our attempts to do so embody descriptive terms which themselves require definition. And, of course, many of our concepts are spatial or take some other non-verbal form. These, like their verbal counterparts, help us adapt to the environment and are the building blocks of thought. Without concepts, we would have no means of attempting to understand the world and ourselves. Possibilities for communication would be severely restricted and our confusion would approach that of Helen Keller before she learned to represent events by touch.

Principles

The term, *principle* embodies the concept of regularities. Principles account for observed regularities of relationship and are thus summarising statements: for example, the principle of reinforcement is a summary statement of the relationship between behaviour and its consequences. This kind of statement, however, can only be made on the basis of careful experiments, such as have been carried out with pigeons in a Skinner box. These experiments, with variables such as hunger, which might influence learning, are controlled, so that the pigeon's pecking performance can with validity be related to variations in reinforcement. Outside the laboratory, the regularity of relationship expressed by the principle may break down. A therapist might find that social reinforcement relates to desirable behaviour for many individuals, but not for those who are withdrawn or psychopathic. Experience will teach her to distinguish between general principles and principles which are applicable in specific situations.

Where regularities of relationship are found, a causal role cannot be ascribed to some variable just because it frequently occurs in conjunction with another. Researchers often describe associations of this kind mathematically, for example as correlations, but correlations do not indicate causes. All that can be said about correlated events is either that one might cause the other, or that both may be caused by some other variable, or by a number of interacting variables. We shall return to the issue of correlation and cause when discussing models of health and illness.

In science, principles that have consistent support are often called 'laws', as when scientists speak of the laws of Boyle or Kepler. The terms do not mean, however, that the cause and effect relationships specified are 'proven'. Even laws of apparently high probability may one day be discounted – a possibility we will illustrate in our discussion of theories. For the moment, it is sufficient to say that principles are the best prevailing statements about a given set of relationships. Within a theoretical framework, they are the elements that guide our reasoning (as when we reason logically) and, indeed, our actions and practice within and outside the field of work.

Theories

It is sometimes thought that theories are the tools of philosophers, innovators and scientists alone, in their efforts to make sense of the world. This view is mistaken. We all use theories in everyday life in attempts to explain events. If, for example, we expect a telephone call which does not come, we postulate theories to explain the event (or non-event in this particular example): perhaps the expected caller misunderstood the agreement, or was taken ill, or has formed a sudden dislike of us. In this case, we have formed a set of hypotheses or theoretical statements – however restricted the content – to explain the circumstance.

Scientific theories

Scientific theories are not really very different from their everyday counterparts. They, too, are presented in statement form, but are generally more informative and are phrased in such a way that their predictions can be tested. A scientific theory is generally concerned with fairly complex issues, and embodies a network of assumptions, constructs and relationships, postulated to explain and predict phenomena; in other words, it is well structured, and its components inter-related, so that either the theory or an auxiliary hypothesis should be able to specify the conditions under which phenomena will or will not occur.

There is a further misconception in our thinking about science which deserves to be raised. This is the misconception that scientific theories are model theories, since they are certain in a way that no others can be. They are not. Scientific knowledge is not certain; nor are the theories which underpin this knowledge by any means certain or true. A brief review of the principal methods of science will bear out this assertion.

Induction and deduction Philosophers have long identified two forms of reasoning which govern scientific advancement: induction and deduction. Induction is said to occur when, on the basis of repeated observations, we proceed to form a general rule. In deduction, on the other hand, we begin by acknowledging that a problem exists and formulating a tentative answer to it. This tentative answer, or hypothesis, is drawn up in the form of a statement and from it we deduce the consequences, or the facts that are likely to follow if the hypothesis is correct. The full name for this method of reasoning is the hypothetico-deductive method.

Bacon For a long time, the accepted position in philosophy was that induction governs scientific development. The case for the inductive method was first argued in detail by Francis Bacon (1561–1626) in 1605 and was elaborated by the British Empiricists. Bacon claimed that what scientists do is gather facts and conduct experiments; on the basis of their observations, they then make generalisations to explain relationships. If these general statements are not disproved, they achieve the status of established laws or theories. In short, Bacon and his followers argued that induction is the method by which true theories are developed.

Hume Ironically, it was an empiricist, David Hume (1711–76) who first threw a spanner in the works of arguments for induction. While Hume held that induction remained the principal method of science, he nevertheless showed that it is impossible to establish the truth of an inductive inference; for no matter how many observations have confirmed it, there always remains the possibility that it may be discounted by some test or observation in the future. Logically, it is clear that induction is an argument from the particular (or a set of particulars) to the general. Such arguments are always fallacious.

Popper A problem arising from Hume's treatment of theories is that of whether theories all are equally acceptable if verification is impossible. This remained a philosophical puzzle until 1959, when the English version of *The Logic of Scientific Discovery* by Karl Popper was published. Popper contends that Hume's problem must be taken seriously, and he agrees that it is impossible to verify a theory. Instead, he argues, theories are developed by the hypothetico-deductive method. A theory is no more than a conjecture or hypothesis, but it generates deductions which can be tested. Although tests can never prove that the theory is true, they can certainly prove it false. The best theories are those which have a high information content: it is this attribute which makes them testable, and therefore *falsifiable*.

Popper's philosophy of science was inspired by the history of science and, in particular, by Einstein's challenge to Newton. Newton's theory of gravity had survived centuries of tests, and scientists were so convinced of its truth that they spoke of his 'laws'. Then Einstein put forward an alternative theory, containing predictions not found in Newton's. These predictions have been confirmed and today Einstein's theory is the best that we have. However, Popper cautions, we can never say that it is true, only that it is an approximation to the truth; it remains the best theory because it has, so far, survived repeated attempts at falsification.

Popper's main concern is to emphasise that theories are not themselves factual, but are merely human explanations of facts and events which must be subject to logical analysis; yet they remain the most powerful tools we have for understanding the world. Through the power of thought alone, Einstein made predictions about the way the universe works, long before the means to test all his predictions were developed: there were no particle accelerators or atomic clocks, let alone satellites, when he first advanced his theories. Outside the physical sciences, our knowledge of human behaviour is likewise grounded in theories. However, it is often difficult to test these with the same precision. For the most part, a complex interaction of variables governs human conduct, and it is this complexity which makes evaluation difficult. Statistical tests allow us to account for the interaction of many variables, but there may be some which are overlooked. Those theories whose predictions are easily tested tend to be unduly reductionist.

Consistency of human behaviour

Investigators of human behaviour recognise that humans are more variable in response than lower order animals, and a great deal more variable than inanimate matter. In a given situation, a group of individuals will seldom respond in exactly the same way; moreover, when the situation is repeated, the same individual may react differently on different occasions. Can we then conclude that human behaviour is totally random and erratic? The answer is an emphatic no. Controlled observations show that if we study sufficiently large samples of people, definite and consistent trends emerge. We can also see trends or tendencies in experimental situations where the samples are quite small. Although it took several replications to establish a pattern, the well-known experiments of Solomon Asch (1952, 1955), in their standard form, used groups of only seven to nine participants, and the focus was on a single 'naive' subject. On the basis of these experiments (conducted, naturally, within a theoretical framework) Asch could declare that social pressure produces conformity. This does not mean that all of his subjects made erroneous judgements all of the time in order to agree with a 'rigged' group consensus. What did happen was that, on average, subjects conformed in one-third of the trials, while 74% conformed at least once. Asch's principle is not, therefore, an absolute one. Basically, it is a statement of what most people do in specified circumstances; that is to say, it specifies a tendency or probable pattern of behaviour which can be analysed statistically.

Social scientists develop theories in the belief that human behaviour is reasonably stable or consistent. They accept that groups are more consistent than individuals, and that the larger the group, the greater the consistency, since in large samples results will not be greatly affected by the vagaries of a few individuals. Within any culture, social research bears out this consistency. It can determine rates and average ages of marriage and death, the number of students entering higher education, and consumption levels of items such as alcohol or heating oil. These trends tend to be fairly stable; they therefore allow quite reliable predictions to be made, say from one year to another, or from one season to the next. A simple prediction would be that people will use more heating oil in winter than in summer. This will not hold good, of course, for all persons, but it is an assertion that can be confirmed or refuted in terms of statistical probability. The assertions of the behavioural sciences are mostly of this nature. In clinical pharmacology, for example, a researcher can say that a drug is effective because it has been successful in treating a large number of people, though not the total sample tested. Likewise, in therapeutic professions, the best treatments are those whose success rates are established, although effectiveness may not be 100% or anything approaching this rate. By using the methods of science – i.e. experimental and control groups, or similar methodology – hypotheses can be accepted if we can show statistically that the results are unlikely to have occurred by chance. Lipsey (1983) calls hypotheses of this kind *statistical hypotheses*, as opposed to *deterministic hypotheses* which admit no exceptions.

It must be admitted that although behavioural scientists speak of established statistical hypotheses, these hypotheses are only provisionally confirmed. We have already discussed Popper's contention that the hypotheses of physical science cannot be verified beyond doubt, since it is always possible that some future event might refute them. The same qualification applies to statistical hypotheses. Our theories to explain what most people do today, or have done in the past, are not so certain that we can predict the future with absolute confidence. We can say what people will probably do, but probability of its nature implies a degree of uncertainty. Even the best informed historians were unable to predict the extraordinary events that occurred in Eastern Europe in 1989. The past, in other words, served as a poor guide to the future. Likewise, our theoretical understanding of disease and its causes was insufficient to predict the AIDS epidemic. Stock-market crashes are further examples of events which hit the unprepared. Indeed, if it were possible to predict even economic trends with confidence, there would be many more very rich people in the world than in fact exist. Our expectation, then, that the future will be much like the past is, as Popper points out, a psychological and not a logical assumption.

Popper   Popper recognises that social theories pose special problems of evaluation. Nevertheless, he argues that if these claim seriously to be scientific, they must contain hypotheses whose predictions can be tested. In the course of his work, Popper has launched a consistent attack on theories which fail in this respect, those of Marx and Adler being favourite targets (e.g. see Popper 1966). He claims that theories of this kind are actually 'pseudoscience', since they interpret every event as verification. By the same token they are also dogmatic, and belong to the realm of metaphysics, not that of science (Popper 1966).

Popper's later work, however, modifies the views presented above (see Popper 1976). Here, he acknowledges that even metaphysical theories can benefit from discussion and review. Just as scientific theories must be testable, Popper proposes that all our theories – philosophical and personal – should be aired for criticism. In this way, they lose their dogmatic quality and become more objective.

For those of us who work within the framework of behavioural and paramedical science, Popper's philosophy offers a challenge. It urges us to adopt a critical attitude to the theories which underlie our work, and presents criticism itself in a positive light. Writing on the theoretical foundations of occupational therapy, Clark (1979) observes that because locale and client problems are so diverse, therapists cannot expect a single theory to guide them in every aspect of professional practice. In these circumstances, the therapist must select from a body of theory only those elements which are relevant to the treatment situation. And where the actual outcome differs from that predicted by the relevant part of the theory, here again a critical attitude is warranted. It may be that the theory is generally false, or that its deductions simply do not fit a given therapeutic situation. The point at issue is that where practitioners feel the need to challenge accepted theory, this is logically admirable if there are genuine grounds for doubt.

Paradigms

The term 'paradigm' has been popularised by Thomas Kuhn, who, like Popper, is an influential philosopher of science. For Kuhn

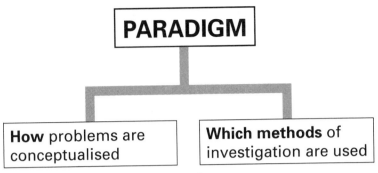

Fig. 1.1 The cognitive function of a paradigm.

(1962), a paradigm is an actual achievement in science which is accepted by the scientific community to the extent that it influences approaches to problems and subsequent research. The cognitive function of a paradigm is to specify how problems are conceptualised and which methods of investigation will be used (Fig 1.1). In physics, light characterised as transverse wave motion is an example of a 19th century paradigm, while, today, light as photons is the paradigm that guides research.

Kuhn has, in fact, employed the term paradigm in a number of ways. Broadly speaking, it denotes on the one hand a model answer to a particular problem – that is, a 'puzzle-solution' and – on the other, the beliefs, values and theories which are shared by members of a scientific community. But Kuhn has used the term in many other senses, a fact he admits in a 1969 postscript to a re-edition of *The Structure of Scientific Revolutions*, originally published seven years earlier. Here, and in his later work (1977) he redefines paradigms as 'exemplars'. In this sense, they show how concrete problems have been approached in the past and so serve as examples for present-day attempts at solution.

In a symposium on the philosophy of science, convened in London in 1965, Kuhn's concept was debated at length.[†] Participants pointed to his inconsistent use of the term, and examined his claim that paradigms guide the progress of what he calls 'normal' science as much as that of 'extraordinary' science – too often the exclusive concern of philosophers. Normal science can be defined as routine,

---

[†] The proceedings of this symposium (or 'colloquium') have been published in four volumes. The fourth volume, *Criticism and the Growth of Knowledge* (Lakatos & Musgrave 1970) is of most relevance to this chapter.

conventional science as practised by possibly the majority of researchers and professionals. Extraordinary science reflects the revolutionary achievements of creative thinkers such as Newton, Einstein, Hawking and Nobel prize winners. Popper's (1970) reply to Kuhn is that 'normal' science indeed exists, but that it has little to recommend it – that it is the activity of the conservative, uncritical professional who hesitates to challenge dogma, and who accepts a new theory only if everyone else is ready to accept it; 'it becomes fashionable by a kind of bandwagon effect'. In Popper's view we ought to feel sorry for Kuhn's 'normal' scientist who has been so badly taught and he elaborates:

I believe, and so do many others, that all teaching on the university level (and if possible below) should be training and encouragement in critical thinking. The 'normal' scientist, as described by Kuhn, has been badly taught. He has been taught in a dogmatic spirit: he is a victim of indoctrination. . . He is, as Kuhn puts it, content to solve 'puzzles'. . . in which a dominant theory (which he calls a 'paradigm') is applied. The success of the 'normal' scientist consists, entirely, in showing that the ruling theory can be properly and satisfactorily applied in order to reach a solution of the puzzle in question.

While Popper consistently makes the point that all our observations are necessarily grounded in theory, he does not agree with Kuhn that theoretical perspectives constitute an orthodoxy which practitioners do not need to challenge. The framework of our assumptions must always be open to criticism, and to accept these frameworks, or paradigms, uncritically is, he claims, to accept the logically mistaken thesis of relativism. He writes of his own position on frameworks that:

I do admit that at any moment we are prisoners caught in the framework of our theories; our expectations; our past experience; our language. But we are prisoners in a Pickwickian sense: if we try, we can break out of our framework at any time. Admittedly, we shall find ourselves again in a framework, but it will be a better and roomier one; and we can at any moment break out of it again.

(Popper 1970, p 56)

While Popper has drawn attention to the logical implications of the concept, paradigm, other writers have observed that the concept is primarily a psychological and sociological one. Thus, Magee (1973) writes that 'Kuhn's theory is in fact a sociological theory about the working activity of scientists in our society.'

If we accept the concept as a sociological one, it describes the advance of science in terms of succession of paradigms (all of which logically remain open to criticism, however well accepted). In this sociological sense, a profession advances when old paradigms are replaced by new ones, which are gradually accepted by its members as more appropriate guides to practice. In the case of occupational therapy, for example, a neuro-behavioural paradigm of man has been replaced by one which takes into account his psychosocial development in addition to his biological inheritance. The older paradigm functions as an exemplar which emphasises treatment at a physical or neuromuscular level. More recent paradigms suggest a broader approach to treatment, and incorporate a number of intervention strategies.

Models

When authors describe the perspectives of a given discipline, they often describe them in the context of a paradigm, as discussed above, or in the context of a model. Since the term, paradigm, contains several different meanings, many authorities prefer to talk of 'models'. A model is a way of representing the natural world in some familiar way, so that our understanding of it may be improved. Models may be specific and physical, or they may take the form of abstract conceptual frameworks. But even physical models have an abstract dimension, since they simplify whatever is represented by abstracting only relevant features.

We are all acquainted with physical or hardware models. These include the model aeroplanes and toy cars of childhood and the models used in our education. We learn anatomy, for example, not only from lectures and textbooks, but also from physical models which represent the human body, or parts of it, such as the heart or liver. Mathematicians, in contrast, use symbolic models, which are highly abstract, or they may use graphs to express correlations or other relationships. Geographers and architects use iconic models (maps and designs), and academic disciplines tend to use theoretical or conceptual models.

Models may be classified according to a number of criteria. A classification by function demarcates descriptive or organising models from predictive kinds, and a classification by form distinguishes between physical, iconic and other types. There are other approaches to classification which need not concern us here. It is more important to address the question of purpose, and it is generally agreed that models have the chief functions shown in Figure 1.2.

Models
Provide framework for complex data
Facilitate visualisation of phenomena
Facilitate communication of ideas
Suggest predictions about the real world and stimulate the development of theories

Fig. 1.2 The chief functions of a model.

Models essentially represent data descriptively, and while they may suggest predictions, they are not required to do so. An adequate theory, on the other hand, is one that makes definite predictions; thus Chorley & Haggett (1967) observe that models and theories cannot be evaluated in similar terms. They note that while we may say that a theory is (provisionally) true, or that it is false, all we can say of a model is that it is appropriate or inappropriate, stimulating or otherwise.

We use models to bring order to the infinite complexities of the world, but our construction of them always involves a simplification of reality, a selectivity of subject-matter, or some undue generalisation. A model, therefore, is never an exact copy of reality, but, rather, provides an analogy to aid our understanding of it.

Models and analogies

Whenever we reason by analogy, we are reasoning on the basis of similarity. This kind of 'as if' reasoning may help us to understand new or unusual problems. Science students, when learning about the concept of force, are often asked to think in terms of Newton's analogy of billiard balls. Likewise, biology textbooks use a lock-and-key analogy or model to illustrate the specific action of enzymes. Perhaps the most dramatic example of successful model building in recent science is that constructed by James Watson and

Francis Crick to represent the structure of DNA. Their approach to the problem was to build several models in the course of their search, until they finally hit upon a double helix structure which 'satisfied both the X-ray data and the laws of stereochemistry' (Watson 1958). This solution, in turn, paved the way for further theoretical developments.

In the sphere of human behaviour, there are many complex processes which are, as yet, not fully understood. In order to provide a framework for these problems, we often construct models, a process which generally involves the use of a more familiar situation as a model for the less familiar. In doing so, we hope that, by analogy, we will understand the second area better if we study its problems in terms of concepts derived from the first. A computer model of the brain, for example, is often used to study thought processes. And, where we do not have clear answers to psychological disorder, we may approach its problems from the framework of a disease model, or perhaps from a mechanistic one which stresses learning as basis for 'maladaptive' behaviour.

Models and theories

Because models are human constructions, they inevitably reflect the culture in which they are developed. Yet they may, at the same time, inspire theories which are independent of their cultural context. The nineteenth century was a time of spectacular advance in physics and chemistry. Its developments inspired Freud's model of man, which saw humans as closed energy systems, bound absolutely by the prevailing principle of determinism. Yet although Freud's model was influenced by the 'Zeitgeist', he developed theories from it which were quite radical by western standards.

Evans (1985) observes that insofar as models are abstract conceptual frameworks, they are 'worldviews' which typically inspire many theories. The relationship between a model and the theories arising from it is, moreover, logical. The 'organismic' model of human nature, for example, is one which portrays the universe as consisting of spontaneously active and developing wholes. The implications of the model focus on autonomy, growth and change, so that a concise prediction of human behaviour is not possible. Theories which are consistent with the organismic model include humanistic theories, and the developmental theories of Erikson and Piaget. Alternatively, a mechanistic model takes a reductionist view of everything in the universe, and focuses on the mechanics of human behaviour as opposed to the whole person. The model im- plies that the behaviour of organisms is determined, and it has inspired the theories of empiricist philosophy and today's behaviourist theories.

Frames of reference

Frames of reference are those aspects of experience which influence our perceptions, decisions and practice. Although human percep- tion is of its nature selective, frames of reference build on this foundation and embody a deliberate orientation to what is relevant. If we are preparing for an examination, for example, we do not study anything and everything. Instead we study within a frame of reference supplied by a syllabus.

In professional practice, a frame of reference serves several func- tions. It specifies the nature, aims and procedures of the work and the features which distinguish it from other forms of practice; it also suggests that some theories are more relevant to practice than others.

Because all forms of practice require an understanding of human beings, there is an inevitable overlap of theory between one thera- peutic profession and another. Thus, psychiatrists, occupational therapists, clinical psychologists, speech therapists and others share, to some extent, a theoretical base. This does not mean, of course, that the professions are equivalent. Each will use, in addi- tion, concepts that are specific to it and that have a particular bearing on treatment procedures. The theoretical base of occu- pational therapy includes concepts relevant to our understanding of man (at neurological, psychological and sociological levels) which may or may not relate to practice. It also includes concepts which relate to assessment and intervention and which give the profession its identity.

Mosey (1970) has written that treatment will ultimately be inad- equate if it is based on an intuitive approach, and that there is little point in using a particular technique simply because others use it, or because it is currently fashionable.* Her plea is for the conscious use of theoretical frames of reference, a plea which the present authors support. Mosey, however, is addressing therapists gener-

---

* Mosey is here objecting to the idea of adhering to a 'paradigm' in the 'exemplar' sense of the word, simply because it happens to be in vogue.

ally, and her discussion of theory includes concepts (e.g. Freudian and Jungian concepts) which are not directly relevant to occupational therapy. She writes that the variety of frames of reference available to therapists is stimulating, and 'allows the therapist to select a frame of reference which is compatible with his values and typical style of interaction' (Mosey 1970, p. 15). In this book, special attention will be paid to the problem of selection. The current theoretical context of practice will be reviewed, making reference, where necessary, to the historical roots of influential ideas. An informed attitude to prevailing theories is clearly important, but this attitude, to be constructive, must also be critical. Therapists cannot, after all, blow with the wind of every fashionable idea. They must remain anchored to the realities of their work, an anchorage which is not necessarily conservative. Frames of reference do, of course, expand and change, but expansion should occur in the context of critical reflection on the profession's nature and purpose.

Criticism and immunisation

While the importance of a critical perspective has been emphasised in this chapter, with particular reference to Popper's views on the matter, it is time to note that Popper has his own critics. Kuhn, as discussed above, objects to Popper's neglect of 'normal science', and others have been critical of his stress on falsification. In the Popperian system, problems precede theories; theories are offered as tentative answers and, if scientific status is claimed for them, they must be falsifiable. A difficulty of this stance is that it is possible, in practice, to defend theories against falsification; that is to say, procedures are available which can be used to protect our basic hypotheses. Generally, these take the form of adding an extra hypothesis or two auxiliary hypotheses to the original theory if it has failed to predict the facts. A theory revised in this way is really an extension of the original one, which, in its new format, is said to be 'immunised'.

Protecting a theory by adding auxiliary hypotheses to it carries the advantage that the theory is not discarded prematurely in the face of contradictory evidence. Newtonian theory, for instance, has failed to yield accurate predictions concerning the motion of a number of planets, yet remains widely used because of its predictive value in non-extreme circumstances. Popper concedes that, provided they are themselves falsifiable, auxiliary hypotheses may add to a theory's scientific content, as happened to Newton's theory following the observed and unpredicted motion of Uranus. On the other hand, he objects to theories whose content is diminished by the addition of endless ad hoc hypotheses and, in this vein, has accused Freud and Marx of reformulating their theories again and again so as to account for every possible eventuality. Taking the view that immunisation has a bearing on how research is conducted, he has commented:

All this suggests the *methodological rule* not to put up with any content-decreasing manoeuvres (or with 'degenerating problem shifts' in the terminology of Imre Lakatos').

(Popper 1976, p 44)

Imre Lakatos, like Popper, worked at the London School of Economics, and has developed his own philosophy of science in which the concept of immunisation plays a major role. Where Kuhn and Popper refer to paradigms and theories respectively, Lakatos refers to conceptual systems as *research programmes*. These may be sociologically successful or otherwise at the level of attracting followers and funding, but they are successful at a rational level only if they cope with more problems than do rival programmes, and add to the store of scientific knowledge.

Research programmes

Methodology

In a lengthy essay on methodology, Lakatos (1970) has proposed that Popper's approach to falsification is relatively naive. Popper, he writes, has failed to note that it is actually impossible to falsify a theory with conviction, since observations aimed at refuting a theory may be inaccurate, or, as Stephen Hawking (1988) has recently pointed out, 'you can always question the competence of the person who carried out the observation'. As an improvement on Popper's thesis, Lakatos proposes one which emphasises protective strategies. He contends that we should not be too critical of the theories which underlie programmes, but should endeavour to save them by making theoretical adjustments in the form of auxiliary hypotheses. Once we have included these, we are in a position where a series of theories are available for scrutiny instead of isolated theories.

The 'hard core'

The procedure recommended by Lakatos is aimed at defending theories against sudden annihilation at the hands of the falsification principle, known in logic as the *modus tollens*. To strengthen the defence, he has introduced a methodological rule or 'negative heuristic', which specifies practices to be avoided. Chiefly, this negative heuristic forbids direction of the falsification principle at what he calls the 'hard core' of a given programme.

Instead, we must use our ingenuity to articulate or even invent "auxiliary hypotheses", which form a *protective belt* around this core, and we must redirect the *modus tollens* to *these*. It is this protective belt of auxiliary hypotheses which has to bear the brunt of tests and get adjusted and re-adjusted, or even completely replaced, to defend the thus-hardened core.

(Lakatos 1970, p 133)

Since, as we shall see in later chapters, the notion of a hard core has been applied to the theoretical base of occupational therapy, Lakatos' use of the concept requires some elaboration. Essentially, he uses the term to describe the basic theories that guide scientific research. These, of course, vary from discipline to discipline, but whatever form they take they should remain unchanged. This stance suggests that Lakatos believes in theoretical certainty. In fact he does not, and, as we have noted, has paradoxically drawn attention to the uncertainty that is inherent in the concept of refutation itself. Having highlighted this and other philosophical difficulties which bestrew the path of the intending researcher, he recognises that some kind of starting point is necessary. We cannot flounder around forever in a sea of doubt, therefore we must accept a stable theoretical core if we are to proceed with the business of science (or, in our case, that of professional practice). Where the researcher is concerned, the decision to adopt a hard core is a strategic one. It is made at the programme's outset and serves to direct attention to issues that should be pursued. Thereafter, the scientist attempts to refute only auxiliary hypotheses; refutation – as Lakatos uses the term – involves pointing to 'anomalies' or 'inconsistencies' between theory and practice.

Although pragmatic considerations enter the picture when the scientist chooses a theoretical core, the selection process is obviously not an arbitrary one. As Lakatos (1970, p 133) puts it, 'The actual hard core of a programme does not actually emerge fully armed like Athene from the head of Zeus. It develops slowly, by a long, preliminary process of trial and error.' There remains the question of whether the hard core is sacrosanct in its own right, or whether it can be replaced. Lakatos allows that it can, since he writes, 'we maintain that if and when the programme ceases to anticipate novel facts, its hard core might have to be abandoned: that is, our hard core . . . may crumble under certain conditions' (Lakatos 1970, p 134). Despite this possibility, he champions a protected theoretical belt whenever possible, quoting the 'greatness' of Newton's programme in support of his position. Newtonian laws of dynamics and gravity formed the theory's hard core, and, by defending these against attack, Lakatos argues, scientists greatly enriched the theory's content at the level of auxiliary hypotheses.

Concluding comments

In this preliminary chapter, we have been faced with a challenging problem – that of attempting to define and describe highly abstract and difficult themes in such a way that educators and postgraduates will find the material of interest, while at the same time not discouraging readers new to the field. Rather than writing in terms so simple as to be judged facile, we decided on a strategy of dealing squarely with theoretical issues, while nevertheless eschewing undue elaboration. Our policy has been one of referring principally to original sources, so that interested readers may go to these for further information. This chapter aims only to furnish the student with the substance of core arguments, and to provide a source of reference, clarifying abstract terms which appear frequently in the text.

It should be noted here that some of the terms we have mentioned can be, and often are, used interchangeably. This is particularly true of the terms *theory*, *model* and *paradigm*. Although a theory generally contains a network of postulates, it may take the form of a series of simple conjectural statements, and can be drawn up without reference to any model or paradigm. As we have seen, models serve to generate theories and are not falsifiable in the same way, since we can only say that they are useful, appropriate or whatever. Theories, models and paradigms are not, then, identical, but there are instances when one term will serve as well as another. Freud's theory is one such instance. In this, man is viewed 'as if' he were a closed energy system, and concepts from the domain of physics are used to explain much of what he does. This, therefore, is a genuine model of man, in that it is undoubtedly grounded in an analogy.* The Freudian account of humankind is also a theory,

---

* By the same criterion, it is evidently less valid to use the term 'humanist model', since the analogy in question is not by any means so clear. Writers who do use this term are probably using the vaguer notion of a model as a 'world view' or 'abstract conceptual framework'.

and it is also a paradigm to the extent that others share the assumptions of psychoanalysis and take Freud's approach to therapy as an 'exemplar' of practice. For these reasons, writers have variously and validly described psychoanalysis as a theory, model or paradigm.

A considerable part of this chapter has focused on philosophical concepts, in particular those from the philosophy of science, because they appear frequently in the professional literature. We have highlighted the nature of theoretical systems because of the inevitable link that exists between how we conceptualise events – professional and otherwise – and how we act.

In the case of the health professions, theoretical perspectives have an important bearing on practice, since they embody values which bear upon our approach to treatment. Allport (1963) has defined a value as 'a belief upon which a man acts by preference' – a definition which presumably includes the values of a woman. What is important about this definition is that it makes clear that there is a definite link between values and action. This claim for a link between perspective, values and professional practice is a theme which runs through the present text.

2. Theoretical perspectives: purpose and relevance to health care

INTRODUCTION: THEORETICAL FRAMEWORKS

Just as scientists use theories, models and paradigms as frameworks for their observations, so we all use frameworks to guide us in our work. Indeed, Piaget (1950) has shown that we interpret events generally in terms of cognitive 'schemata', whether or not these pertain to work. This chapter will be concerned with the link that exists between theory and therapeutic procedure. The history of health care is one in which perspective and practice have intermingled over the years, and this will be illustrated by selected examples. The theories reviewed at this stage are not necessarily directly compatible with occupational therapy. Traditions and philosophies that are specific to the profession will be reviewed in the next chapter; in the meantime, we will address the broader question of how theories may relate, and have related in the past, to forms of therapeutic practice. The account which follows makes it clear that theoretical perspectives are never static. Like Piaget's schemata, they develop and change in order to incorporate or accommodate to new data.

Prescientific theories

Many thousands of years ago, Stone Age man evidently believed that atypical behaviour indicated possession by evil spirits. This perspective led to a primitive, but curiously logical, form of treatment for headaches, convulsions and other sicknesses. A 'cure' was effected by using chisels made of stone to create an opening in the skulls of afflicted persons. This opening, called a trephine, allowed the evil spirits to escape.

Magical thinking and demonology coloured approaches to illness up to and beyond the Christian epoch. Even in the New Testament, there are references to devils and 'unclean' spirits which take over the bodies of their unfortunate victims. However, primitive thinking at this stage had been modified to some extent by Hippocrates (460–357 B.C.), the philosopher and physician who, by common agreement, is the founder of modern medicine. He protested at the barbaric punishments and floggings that were used to discourage inhabiting demons, and related mental disorders to physical causes, with emphasis on brain pathology.

With the decline of Greek and Roman civilization, the scientific approach to medicine inspired by Hippocrates waned in Europe. During the Middle Ages, unusual disorders – in particular those of a psychological nature – were once again related to demonic possession. However, this time, a new dimension was added. Disordered individuals were thought to be witches who had made a pact with the devil. Persecution, torture and burning of these 'witches' was the order of the day.

The Renaissance saw the re-emergence of a scientific perspective. In London, the College of Physicians received its charter from Henry VIII in 1518, and there followed a proliferation of hospitals, asylums and scientific bodies over the next two centuries. Alongside these developments, however, questionable theories continued to influence very doubtful practices. During the seventeenth century, the belief that illnesses of all sorts could be cured by purging the system was rampant. Doctors used emetics, purgatives and blood letting with enthusiasm, and, indeed, these practices carried over to the eighteenth century. George III, who ascended the English throne in 1760, was subjected to horrific rituals of blood letting in attempts to cure his mental instability – now thought to have been due to porphyria. Quackery, with its paraphernalia of leeches, cuppings and the like, finally yielded to the scientific advances which followed.

Dualism and reductionism

Approaches to treatment grew less superstitious over the centuries, but came instead to be influenced by *dualist* philosophy, whose origins can be traced to the French philosopher, René Descartes (1596–1650). Descartes proposed that the universe operates like a huge machine whose mechanics can be understood with certainty through investigating its parts. His view of human beings was that a thinking mind inhabits a machine-like body. Interaction between the two is minimal and neither one can influence the other. Since the body was conceived of as a machine, within a mechanistic universe, Descartes proposed that its operations should be studied without reference to the mind. Under the influence of Cartesian philosophy, physicians divided into two camps: those who treated the mind in its own right, and those who treated the body without reference to the mind. To consider that the body is governed by laws which exclude mental influences is a form of what is known as a *reductionist* position. Reductionism is at the heart of two influential, although questionable, models of behaviour which relate to health and disorder: the biomedical and the behaviourist models. Reference will be made to these models in due course. For the present, we shall merely note that proponents of a holistic perspective are, naturally, highly critical of reductionist approaches to treatment, together with the mechanistic model of humankind that they entail. Nowadays, we are ever more aware that Chinese and other traditions of health-care have always acknowledged the totality of the person, whereas western medicine lost this insight in the course of its development. This awareness coincides with current pleas for a return to a holistic perspective on human nature, and this perspective is indeed growing in influence. Today, it is most closely identified with humanistic psychology. Since this movement arose, in part, as a protest against psychoanalysis, the psychoanalytic perspective is outlined below.

The psychoanalytic perspective

Freud

Psychoanalysis – as both a theory and a form of treatment – was originated by Sigmund Freud (1856–1939). The context of prevailing ideas in which Freud developed this theory included the concepts of nineteenth century physics, and those of Charles Darwin. Accordingly, Freudianism incorporates concepts pertaining to mankind's striving for survival (Eros or the 'life instinct') and to the conservation of energy (the interplay between id, ego and superego, and the idea of catharsis). The influence of contemporary ideas is further seen in Freud's adoption from physics of the concept of determinism, and, from the social sciences, the idea that humankind's behaviour is governed by instincts, unconscious or otherwise. Given his initial commitment to the view that the life instinct governs our efforts to survive against the odds, it is of relevance to the ideas expressed in the previous chapter that

Freud had to revise his theory in the face of some observations to the contrary. For example, the idea of a life instinct is hardly compatible with the observed facts that some people indulge in masochistic behaviour, or become depressed, or commit suicide. Thus, Freud added the auxiliary hypothesis of a death instinct to his initial theory.

As a total system, psychoanalysis provides a clear example of the relationship between theory and therapeutic practice. A central tenet is that neurotic disorders are rooted in conflict, a condition which arises when people protect themselves from anxiety by avoiding recognition of their fears and real motivations. This means that, according to Freud, psychic energy is bound up in keeping conflict at bay. Less energy is therefore available to the rational ego.

Psychoanalytic therapy endeavours to restore full awareness of conflicts denied access to consciousness. It is assumed that because defence mechanisms (repression and so forth) operate to keep awareness at bay, the client cannot simply tell the therapist what the root of the trouble is. Free association and dream symbol analysis are therefore used to bypass self-censorship.

Relevance to practice

The question of whether psychoanalytic principles are relevant to the practice of occupational therapy is an important one. Regarding this issue, Kielhofner & Burke (1983) write that, for a time, psychoanalysis *did* influence the profession. Therapists used crafts and activities as a means of investigating unconscious material, and Mosey (1970) has described the development of an art test battery, adapted for psychiatric occupational therapy. On the basis of interview and test performance, she writes, (p 70), 'the therapist attempts to identify the various complexes which are disturbing the patient'. Again, on the theme of symbolism and object-relations analysis, Mosey observes that the tools and materials of therapy often become symbols of unconscious processes. She quotes the example of a girl engaged in woodwork for whom the chisel had 'evident' sexual significance, and whose gentle rubbing of oil into the wood symbolised a yearning for nurturing.

In the rational climate of modern psychology, symbolic interpretations of this kind are rare indeed and, where they do exist, remain the province of convinced psychoanalysts. They are certainly unlikely to play any great role in occupational therapy in the future. Barris, Kielhofner & Watts (1983) explain the influence of psychoanalysis in terms of pressure brought to bear on occupational therapists by psychiatrists of Freudian persuasion. They note criticism of its influence by therapists, who feel that it marks an unjustified departure from the profession's original mission, and a misuse of activity whose main purpose is the promotion of adaptive behaviour. They add (p 27) that 'it appears that classic psychoanalysis has little in common with occupational therapy'.

In view of the above comments, it is logical to query the incorporation of psychoanalytic theory into so many curricula. One might as well query, however, the inclusion of medicine and surgery, since occupational therapists are not doctors and will never perform surgical operations. Although psychoanalytic principles are not directly relevant to practice, they may usefully extend our appreciation of human nature. To know that people may use defence mechanisms in the face of illness, addiction and threat furthers our understanding, patience and sympathy. Freud's contribution to all forms of therapy should also be acknowledged, in that it was he who established the primacy of the one-to-one therapeutic encounter. Furthermore, Freud never accepted dualism. His insistence that the relationship between mind and body is one of reciprocal influence underpins current thinking on psychosomatic disorder.

The psychoanalytic model and determinism

Although it is not dualist, psychoanalysis *is* deterministic. Influenced as he was by the physics of his day, Freud applied the principle of determinism to a wide range of human experience. His concept of man includes the claim that man is dominated by instincts, that instincts have psychological and physical components, and that they often motivate us unconsciously. Since all human actions have motivational roots, whether or not they are consciously acknowledged, it follows that everything we do is determined, nothing is random. As is well known, Freud believed that even jokes, dreams and slips of the tongue have hidden causes.

There is an anomaly in Freud's theory that is often overlooked: for all its determinism, the theory contains the possibility that after psychoanalysis the individual has a new freedom of choice. Technically, this is due to the redirection of psychic energy, which is now placed at the disposal of the rational, goal-choosing ego. Having gained insight into the circumstances of his life, pschoanalysed man, freed from conflict and mature in self-knowledge, is now ready to face the world anew. But this development is due wholly to therapy. Freud's vision of the human condition generally remains one in which possibilities for self-determination are deemed to be severely restricted. This aspect of his theory and his alleged emphasis on biological motivating forces have come under attack, during and after his lifetime.

Challenges to psychoanalysis have taken many forms, and there have been several modifications of the system. These include the development of neo-Freudian theories and a host of alternative therapies. One of the most influential challenges has been that posed by humanistic psychology, at both theoretical and therapeutic levels.

The humanistic perspective

Humanism has always been associated with concepts of personal freedom, self-determination and creativity. It is an optimistic vision of mankind's potential that has waxed and waned through various epochs of history. It inspired a great deal of early Greek art and architecture and, centuries later, the achievements of the Renaissance. Today, the perspective is associated with several theories in philosophy, chiefly those which embrace existentialism, but its influence on psychology is relatively recent. Humanistic psychology and existentialist theories have much in common, but they are by no means identical. The historical roots of each perspective have been traced by Cracknell (1984), writing specifically for occupational therapists, and so will not be discussed again here. Neither will the vast number of psychological theories that have been influenced by the humanistic movement be elaborated. Instead, the contribution of two important protagonists, Abraham Maslow and Carl Rogers is discussed, concentrating on their central concepts.

Maslow

Maslow's questioning of prevailing paradigms began in the 1950s, although it was not until 1968 that he published his influential book, *Towards a Psychology of Being*. In the meantime, he was at work on other publications in which he developed his objections to the orthodoxy of the day and began to propose alternative ways of looking at human beings. He attacked psychoanalysis for its focus on the neurotic aspects of personality, and for its determinism. Likewise, he attacked the determinism of behavioural theory, in particular its central concept that all behaviour is 'conditioned'.

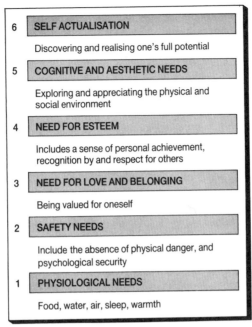

Fig. 2.1 Maslow's hierarchy of needs (reproduced from Creek J (ed) 1990 Occupational therapy and mental health. Churchill Livingstone, Edinburgh).

The essence of Being, according to Maslow, is not that we are buffeted by instinct and drives, nor that we can be characterised by conditioned reflexes. Rather, we are whole, free, healthy and purposeful. He proposed a new focus on this wholeness of personality, and turned himself to the study of healthy, well-functioning individuals.

Motivation is a core concept in Maslow's philosophy. While he does not dispute the reality of the needs and drives outlined by other psychologists, he does dispute the claim that they are the prime motivators. His alternative conceptualisation is that motives form a hierarchy (Fig. 2.1). At the bottom of the hierarchy are basic needs, such as physiological and safety needs. Naturally, these play a role in human behaviour, but Maslow points out that these are, in fact, in large part met – at least in the more developed countries of today. In his view, basic needs motivate us only when they are not adequately met; once they are, the next group of needs in the hierarchy becomes influential until they, in turn, are satisfied. At the top of the hierarchy is the self-actualisation motive, the motive which demands of us that we become fully human, fully ourselves. It is a striving which, according to Maslow's own investigations, characterises the most mature and healthy individuals in our society, and which has been summed up in the dictum: 'What man can be, he must be'. In 1970, Maslow gave a more complete definition of self-actualisation as 'the full use and exploration of talents, capacities, potentialities'.

Rogers

Carl Rogers, like Maslow, believes that humans are essentially free and capable of transcending the limitations placed upon them. As a psychology graduate with an interest in psychotherapy, it became clear to him that existing practices were flawed. Specifically, he objected to the view that, in therapy, one person, the therapist, gives an objective account of whatever is wrong with the other, the 'patient'. Rogers believes that the therapist does not 'cure' the 'patient'. Rather, the 'client' is capable of change and growth of his own accord, and the therapist merely tries to facilitate this process. It is not up to the therapist to make so-called objective judgements about the client, but to understand his way of looking at the world and at himself. This Rogerian emphasis on the reality of subjective experience and the phenomenological self shows how much the theory is influenced by existentialism. Maslow's influence is also evident. Rogers acknowledges the self-actualising tendency as the dominant one in human experience. This underlies the organism's striving for autonomy and self enhancement.

Since the humanistic account of humankind describes people in terms that are highly positive and optimistic, the cynical reader might wonder why individuals ever present at therapy in the first place. The answer is that the growth process natural to man may be temporarily blocked – a possibility that Rogers also attempts to explain.

Rogers' account of the above possibility invokes some principles of development, chiefly those that pertain to development of the self-concept. His account notes that the striving for self-enhancement requires, in the first instance, a positive 'condition of worth'. Yet he notes that if we are to feel positive about ourselves, this requires that parents and other adults also see us in an affirmative light. But all too often parents value their children on an 'if' basis. Children may be told that they are valued only if they are well-behaved, obedient and fulfilling of adult expectations. The result is that the person's fundamental need for *unconditional positive regard* is thwarted. The outcome of this circumstance is as follows: the individual strives for self-enhancement, but at the same time strives to gain self-regard on the conditional terms set by another. Then, at some point, the incompatibility of these expectations comes to the fore. This incompatibility is not acknowledged consciously. In Rogerian terms, the person is now experiencing 'incongruence' – the vague feeling that there is a discrepancy between the life one is actually leading and the concept of self. In short, incongruence refers to a discrepancy between self and experience, and the individual who is experiencing incongruence is actually unconsciously asking the question: 'How can I please others and also myself while remaining an integrated human being?'

Client-centred therapy The Rogerian approach to therapy centres on the belief that individuals have within themselves their own resources for improvement. As we have already noted, Rogers believes that the therapist's role is at best a facilitating one. The therapist endeavours to create conditions in which the client feels free to explore problems of incongruence by offering him or her *acceptance*, *respect* and *empathy* (Fig. 2.2). Where necessary, he or she reflects the client's own feelings and attitudes, so that the client can better analyse the problems in question and move more easily toward a solution. Above all, the client-centred therapist offers the *unconditional positive regard* that may be missing in the person's life. It is hoped that by this means people will talk more honestly about themselves, and that by virtue of the therapist listening to what is said and encouraging self-expression, feelings will be clarified and

Therapist offers:
Unconditional positive regard
Acceptance
Respect
Empathy

Fig. 2.2 Client-centred therapy.

insight achieved. This client-centred approach is often called *non-directive therapy*.

Relevance to practice

As is the case with psychoanalysis, the client-centred approach does not have a direct bearing on the practice of occupational therapy. After all, the person presenting for treatment is not seeking some form of verbal therapy which he can gain elsewhere: he is, rather, seeking some form of activity which has a therapeutic aim, and which is specific to the therapy's intervention procedures. Nevertheless, in the broad sense of the term, the humanistic perspective is of prime importance in that it can inform our professional outlook. If we are persuaded by it, we will perceive the person we are treating, first and foremost as a human being; other roles – such as the 'patient' role – become of incidental concern, and, in acknowledging the client's humanity, we are also acknowledging the active and positive contribution he makes to treatment. The therapeutic process, in these terms, becomes one of shared responsibility.

Chapter 3 lists some values that, by agreement, govern the occupational therapist's perception of her role. It will be clear that these are nothing if not humanistic.

The medical perspective

The medical approach to health care is too well-known to require any detailed discussion. In the most general sense, it is concerned with the diagnosis and treatment of disease, but it remains highly influenced by the mechanistic model of man introduced by Descartes. While the model has inspired science generally and the biological sciences in particular, it has important limitations. In a comment on these, Capra (1983, p 47) writes:

The problem is that scientists, encouraged by their success in treating living organisms as machines, tend to believe that they are nothing but machines. The adverse consequences of this reductionist fallacy have become especially apparent in medicine, where the adherence to the Cartesian model of the human body as a clockwork has prevented doctors from understanding many of today's major illnesses.

He points out that in terms of Descartes' analogy, a sick person was likened to a clock whose parts were not functioning properly, and that, as medicine advanced under its influence, attention came to focus on the non-functioning parts to the neglect of the whole person.

In summary, the biomedical tradition holds that disorder entails a breakdown in the machinery of the body, which can be put right by applying specific and appropriate physical remedies. When the same approach is applied to the treatment of mental problems, the account given tends to employ the same terms as are used to describe physical illness (Fig. 2.3). The influence of the biomedical model is thus very clear, and although many forms of mental disorder have no known physical cause, they are traditionally treated by physical or chemical means. The analogy inherent in the model is accepted quite literally, and the person treated 'as if' he were ill.

Institutionalised medicine

Although the medical approach is undoubtedly reductionist, few critics would deny medicine's very real achievements. Drugs and immunisation procedures have curtailed many life-threatening diseases, medicine has helped increase the human lifespan, and advances in surgery have brought hope and renewed capacity to many. But these achievements carry their disadvantages. Public expectations are often quite unrealistic. The successes of medicine apply to a restricted range of disorders, yet people expect it to cure them of everything. And the more they expect this, the more

Mental problems
Patient
Presenting symptoms
Aetiology
Incidence
Diagnosis
Treatment
Prognosis

Fig. 2.3 Medical perspective: terms used.

the profession expands: hospitals, regulations, technology and specialists proliferate as medicine becomes more and more institutionalised.

Illich The best known and most vocal critic of institutionalised medicine is undoubtedly Ivan Illich. Over the years, he has been critical of several modern institutions, including schools, on the grounds that they rob individuals of autonomy. Furthermore, he claims, most of today's institutions have reached a point where they have become counterproductive: they are already beginning to crumble under the weight of the demands they have created. In *Medical Nemesis* (1976), Illich writes that people in modern society have forfeited responsibility for their own health. We no longer, he says, decide for ourselves if we are ill, but need a doctor to deliver such a basic verdict. And where a diagnosis of ill-health is made, he continues, we passively hand ourselves over as objects awaiting repair. While he is not alone in condemning reductionist approaches to disorder, Illich's attack is by far the most scathing.

The core of the argument in 'Medical Nemesis' is that whereas older, advisory forms of medicine did not detract from personal responsibility, modern forms create a harmful dependency. In consequence, we succumb all too easily to prescribed treatment, treatment which in turn can actually make us ill. The successes of medicine proceed in tandem with misdiagnosis, drugs that have dangerous side-effects, botched operations and unnecessary surgery. Medicine does not cure us according to Illich: it makes us sicker. We have already noted that medical discoveries have added to the human lifespan, but Illich denies even this. He contends that improvements in health and in life-expectancy rates are due more to improved hygiene and better living conditions, than to the effects of antibiotics and similar drugs.

Many of the ideas expressed by Illich grew out of his experience as a pastor in Latin America. There, he became aware of gross inequities in the social system and the failure of institutions to provide a remedy. He writes that institutions, of their very nature, cannot provide this. As they grow, administrative and research costs spiral, and the individual gets lost in the process of expansion – including the person who most deserves help. Of course, medical programmes are set up in the belief that costs will in time decrease as the nation grows healthier and fewer demands are placed on the system. However, this has seldom if ever been known to happen. Institutional growth creates insatiable consumer demand, and the system becomes overloaded once it passes the point of 'optimal' use of technology. In the final analysis, Illich claims, the 'medicalisation' of health ranks second only to malnutrition in the human damage it causes.

Coleman It has been said that Illich makes dramatic accusations, but offers no solution other than pleading for a return of health care to the individual as his own responsibility. Since his protest, medical technology has continued to advance, and a recent review of current trends has been offered by Coleman (1988) who is himself a medical doctor. In *The Health Scandal*, he claims that medicine today is primarily geared to serving the interests of practitioners, pharmaceutical companies and manufacturers of equipment. This diversion of resources towards technology and away from people is, he argues, wasteful and counterproductive: 'We can no longer afford to spend time and effort on high-technology diagnostic equipment. We need to spend time and effort on helping people'. (p 213). His general thesis is that 'society is becoming sicker and sicker every year' (Box 2.1).

Box 2.1   Coleman's arguments

1. Intensive care units are often unnecessary, and are therefore wasteful of resources. American studies have shown that only 10% of people admitted to these units actually make use of the technology available there. In May 1987, an article in the British Medical Journal showed that heart attack victims have a better chance of survival if they are cared for in a local cottage hospital than they have in a centralised intensive care unit.*

2. 90% of X-rays are unnecessary – as are the majority of tests performed routinely in hospital. Far too many people are therefore exposed to radiation without reason.

3. There are more coronary care units, more cardiologists, more surgical and transplantation techniques than ever before. Nevertheless, record numbers are dying of heart disease. Diabetes, arthritis and other diseases are also on the increase.

4. 80% of people who seek medical help do not need medical treatment, but are treated just the same. Because dangerous drugs are frequently prescribed at random, one

in every ten hospital beds are occupied by people whom medicine has made sick.

5. Advances in medicine do not increase the human lifespan. There is little difference in this respect between nations with high health-care budgets (and therefore higher doctor/patient ratios and hospital bed quotas) and those with relatively low levels of expenditure. In Jamaica, a third-world, low-budget country, the life expectancy for males is 69.2 years. The comparable rates for America and France are 71.8 years and 70.2 years respectively, despite the vast resources these countries devote to health.

6. The more public resources are diverted to medicine, the more people actually become ill, or at least feel they ought to be unwell. Coleman reports a British study in which 95% of the people surveyed believed they had been ill in a given fortnight. One out of every three people believed they were suffering from some long-term illness or disability.

7. Health improves when doctors go on strike. When this happened in Los Angeles in 1976, the death rate fell by 18%. In Israel, where doctors went on strike for a month in 1973, there was a 50% drop in the death rate.

8. Medical research gobbles up funds. Every 28 seconds a new scientific paper is published, and more has been spent on research in the past 20 years than in all previous years added together. Millions of dollars and pounds are spent annually on cancer research, yet the incidence of cancer continues to grow. The profession chases elusive 'magic' cures; meanwhile, the public remains negligent in self-care.

---

* Coleman's referencing system is inconsistent. Sometimes sources are quoted by title and date, sometimes by author(s) and date. For this reason, we refer the reader only to his own text.

Coleman argues that medicine is misdirected in its search for ever more evasive cures. Many modern diseases are man-made, and the associated risk factors (smoking, obesity, toxic chemicals and the like) are all too well known. Yet people are reluctant to act on this knowledge for the sake of their own health. Medicine itself has failed to encourage self-care, for reasons not unconnected with commerce and scientific prestige. It is now time to change and make good the absurd neglect of preventative education.

Our critique of conventional medicine has focused for the most part on its relation to the physical health of communities, and we have said little about its bearing on psychological well-being. Coleman observes that its record here is no better than in other areas. The incidence of major psychiatric disorders has not diminished and, worst of all, psychiatry has had little impact on suicide rates. He quotes several statistics to this effect, including one showing that 66% of suicide cases had visited a doctor within four weeks of death, obviously to no avail. And a favoured method of killing oneself is to use medically prescribed pills. Moreover, doctors themselves commit suicide more than does any other occupational category, according to the (British) Office of Population Censuses and Surveys. Evidence, then, does not seem to corroborate the view that the medical approach to psychological problems is necessarily the best one.

The medical model of psychological disorder

The medical model is one in which the principles of physical medicine are applied to the diagnosis and treatment of atypical behaviour. It focuses on assumed physiological causes and is therefore reductionist and, indeed, more Cartesian than Descartes ever was. While Descartes proposed a distinction between mind and matter, he never denied the reality of the mind. Yet a great deal of modern psychiatry reduces mind to body and holds that 'mental illness' is essentially a byproduct of some organic pathology.

The idea that mental illness is analagous to physical illness is at the heart of the medical model, as is the related idea that psychiatric patients should be treated 'as if' they were physically ill. In our review of the model, we shall see that it has had its successes and failures over the decades, and that its failures may well be due to taking the analogy inherent in the model far too literally.

Kraepelin

The instigator of the biomedical approach to abnormal behaviour was Emil Kraepelin (1856–1926). At the turn of the century, he proposed that psychiatric disorders are 'diseases' of some sort, and that all are rooted in endocrine or metabolic disturbance. He stressed the part played by heredity, and discounted the possible contribution of psychological and social factors. His main concern, however, was with diagnosis. He believed that this would be made easier if mental illnesses (or 'diseases') were clearly distinguishable one from the other, and he drew up a system of classification which became a model for future developments. This system described the signs and symptoms which tended to occur together in various disorders, and its development helped practitioners to classify or 'diagnose' the presenting behaviour.

Kraepelin's system was welcomed by his contemporaries. He was seen to have brought order where a fair degree of vagueness had previously existed, and to have furnished psychiatrists with well-defined guidelines for practice. However, Kraepelin's chief professional legacy was his advocacy of the existence of a physiological basis to mental disorder. This perspective retains its influence because of its apparent scientific status, and because several hypotheses developed from his biomedical model have been corroborated.

'Organic' disorders: the search for physical causes

Following several discoveries in the twentieth century, the term 'organic' was applied to disorders which relate to brain injury or infection, or to a neurological degenerative process, such as occurs in Alzheimer's disease and Huntington's chorea. With respect to infection, perhaps the most important discovery was that general paresis, and its accompanying mental confusion, is caused by syphilis. It was further found that Huntington's chorea is genetically transmitted, as are many metabolic disorders, such as phenylketonuria (PKU). The identification of PKU was, in fact, due to the persistent efforts of a Norwegian mother who is a model of 'non-passivity'. Refusing to take 'no' or 'I don't know' for an answer, she pursued a succession of doctors for an explanation of her child's mental retardation and unusual odour. Eventually, early in the 1930s, one doctor found excessive phenylpyruvic acid in the child's urine, and pursued its cause. As is now well-known, PKU occurs when the infant lacks the enzyme that metabolises phenylalanine. If this lack is undetected, phenylpyruvic acid builds up in the blood and damages the brain. Today, potential damage is mitigated by placing the child on a phenylalanine-free diet until myelination of neurons is completed.

Although the ravages of most organic conditions cannot, as yet, be either prevented or reversed, the successes outlined above increased medical scientists' faith in the physiological perspective. Yet there remained disorders which fitted uncomfortably into this position; in particular, schizophrenia and severe depression posed problems, as there were difficulties in finding tangible causes. These conditions and their postulated subcategories have been named and re-named in various systems of classification, but whether they are labelled *reactions, illnesses, disorders* or '*functional* psychoses', an exact explanation of their origins remains elusive. This failure to locate a physiological cause naturally poses problems for a strict physiological perspective. Kraepelin's belief that psychosocial factors play no contributing part has not been borne out by the evidence, and genetic influences, for which he made such strong claims, do not tell the whole story. Currently, adherents of the medical model acknowledge non-organic influences but live in the hope that one day a biological cause will be discovered. Meanwhile, victims of schizophrenia and manic-depressive reactions (since 1980, better known as 'bipolar' disorders) are treated 'as if' their condition had a corroborated physical basis.

The medical model of mental disorder has generated several assumptions that have a bearing on diagnosis and treatment, for example:

- that there is a strong hereditary basis to 'functional' disorders (that is, those whose origins have not yet been established)
- that these disorders have chemical or neurological causes
- that physical and chemical methods of treatment are the most appropriate.

Of course, all these assumptions centre on the notion that what is being treated is actually an illness, the illness in question being identified on the basis of a cluster of atypical behaviours which are said to constitute a syndrome.

Investigating the heredity thesis: family and twin studies

While, up to the end of the 1950s, there were grounds for favouring the hypothesis of a genetic explanation of functional disorders, current thinking is that early studies overestimated the genetic component. Research on the issue addresses the question of whether psychiatric disorder occurs more frequently among blood relatives than among people who have no genetic relationship, the majority of studies focusing on identical and non-identical twins. Many of these have been carried out, only a sample can be referred to here.

Percentage

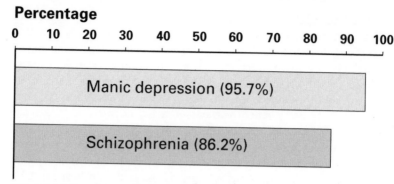

Fig. 2.4   Kellman's concordance rates in identical twins.

The classical twin studies were carried out by Kallman in the 1950s. Long a champion of the heredity cause, he found (1958) that identical twins showed a concordance rate of 95.7% for manic-depressive reactions, and 86.2% for schizophrenia (Fig. 2.4); the rates for dizygotic twins in each case were no higher than those for siblings. However, Kallman's research contained methodological flaws that exaggerated agreement rates. Davison & Neale (1986) have shown that many subsequent studies produced much lower rates. One reason for the discrepancy is that investigators do not always agree on what constitutes concordance. One investigator might decide that the twin of a diagnosed schizophrenic is showing evidence of suspicion amounting to paranoia, while another might put a similar 'symptom' down to acceptable nervousness at being interviewed.

In a study of admissions to a London hospital, Gottesman & Shields (1982) accepted that loose definitions of concordance exaggerate agreement rates, and they established a more stringent criterion. Concordance was agreed on only when a person who was diagnosed for schizophrenia and hospitalised had a twin who met the same conditions. Under these conditions, they found a concordance rate for 24 pairs of monozygotic twins of 42%, falling to 9% for 33 dizygotic pairs (Fig. 2.5). They found, too, that for relatives, the risk of developing the same disorder if one parent is schizophrenic is 13%; the risk for siblings 10%; and that for a nephew or niece, 3% (Fig. 2.6). Other studies have found that adopted children whose natural mothers are schizophrenic are more likely than adopted controls to have schizophrenia, or some other psychiatric disorder, diagnosed in later life (e.g. Heston 1966).

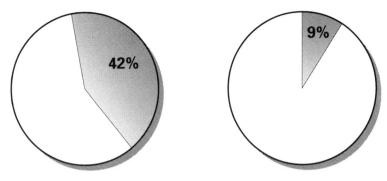

Fig. 2.5 Concordance rate for twins where both of each pair have been diagnosed as suffering from schizophrenia (Gottesman & Shields 1982).

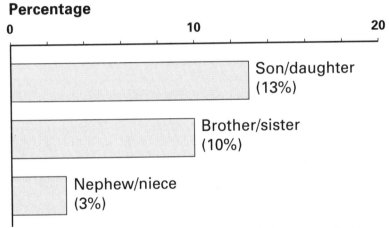

Fig. 2.6 Risks for relatives of developing schizophrenia (Gottesman & Shields 1982).

Neurological and biochemical correlates

CAT scan studies have found that some schizophrenics show signs of brain pathology, as do a number of other people with psychoses of one kind or another. CAT scans typically reveal enlarged ventricles and a lesser degree of cortical atrophy (Weinberger et al 1983). However, since these features are not specific to schizophrenia, and since they characterise only a proportion of sufferers, they are of little use in diagnosis. In efforts to be more precise about the physiological basis of schizophrenia, other investigators have looked for biochemical causes.

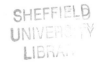

The search for a biochemical explanation of schizophrenia is as old as its history. Once or more in every decade, some researchers come up with a posited chemical solution, such as occurred after the famous 'pink spot' tests of 1962 (Friedhoff & van Winkle). Too often, these studies have not been replicable, or it has been found that the results claimed can be traced to some other factor, for example to hospital diet, stress or treatment procedures. Despite these difficulties, current research has come up with new and interesting biochemical hypotheses. One such hypothesis is that schizophrenia is caused by an excess of the neurotransmitter, dopamine. Dopamine production is increased when amphetamines are administered, so that people who take high doses show schizophrenic-like behaviour. Also, schizophrenics who are given low doses show an increase in symptoms (Snyder 1980). In similar vein, it has been suggested that two neurotransmitters, norepinephrine and serotonin, play a role in affective disorder. Low levels of either one are said to underlie depression, and high levels to be associated with elation.

There are, however, problems with these findings. The results mentioned do not hold good in all instances. For example, amphetamines do not worsen all schizophrenic symptoms; indeed, they even improve symptoms in some cases (Kammen et al 1977). Again, while biochemical differences between psychotic patients and controls may be *correlates* of a particular disorder, we cannot say that they are *causes* of the disorder any more than we can say that fatty deposits on the liver *cause* cirrhosis. In cirrhosis, fatty deposits form *part* of the disease itself and the cause is something quite different, relating to the ingestion of some toxic substance, such as alcohol.

Social influences

In our review of family studies, we saw that the one by Gottesman & Shields (1982) is a model of its kind in that it takes into account difficulties in defining concordance. According to this study, the real concordance rates for schizophrenia among identical twins is 42%. This figure is much higher than the figure for dizygotic twins, and much higher again for those of lesser relationship. Some kind of genetic basis is, therefore, indicated, but the study also points to the contribution of environmental factors. That social class plays a part in schizophrenia has been acknowledged by many (e.g. Strauss 1982), while other investigators have pointed to family pathology (Singer & Wynne 1963, Goldstein 1985). For this reason, recent classifications of psychiatric disorder are less oriented to physical symptoms than formerly. For example, the 1980 Diagnostic and Statistical Manual (DSM-III), published in the United States, offers both diagnostic categories, and also rating-scales for psychosocial stressors, which should be taken into account when making a diagnosis. While the medical model now acknowledges these stressors, it remains focused on biological 'predispositions' and on physical methods of treatment. It has been argued that in view of research findings this focus is illogical, and that the history of psychiatric treatment procedures is not altogether a happy one.

Treatment procedures

In the early part of this century, a variety of therapies were used to treat severely disturbed behaviour. With respect to the psychological approach, psychoanalysis was used with mixed success. On the whole, it appeared most useful as a way of helping 'neurotic' clients, and only a few practitioners used it successfully to treat schizophrenia. It is hard to escape the conclusion that the charisma of the practitioner played no small part in effecting positive outcomes. With respect to physical methods, the first half of the century saw several new developments. Of these, the most widely used procedures were insulin coma treatment, psychosurgery and electroconvulsive therapy. All of these have side-effects of some kind, and, while modifications of them are still in use today, they are less frequently employed than formerly. This is due in part to objections both to the side-effects mentioned and to the unpleasantness of the procedures themselves; but it is mainly due to the development of drug therapy procedures.

Insulin coma treatment Insulin coma treatment, sometimes called insulin shock treatment, was introduced by Manfred Sakel in the 1930s. As the term suggests, the patient is given large doses of insulin to reduce blood sugar levels; he then loses consciousness and falls into a deep coma. It was claimed that, on awakening, the patient became surprisingly lucid, and the procedure was popular for a time. But it contains obvious dangers, such as the production of irreversible coma, and gradually it fell into disrepute.

Psychosurgery In 1936, Egas Moniz introduced the procedure known as prefrontal lobotomy or leucotomy, in the wake of his attendance at a conference where the procedure had been shown to be effective in reducing frustration in chimpanzees. Originally, in its application to humans, two small holes were drilled in the skull so that the nerve fibres connecting the frontal lobes and thalamus could be severed. In subsequent 'improvements' to the technique, entry was achieved through the bony part of the eye socket. Lobotomies were said to be effective to the extent that, after operation, there is a reduction in tension, anxiety and morbid pre-occupations. But this is achieved at a price. To one degree or another, the postoperative patient becomes listless and indifferent to his surroundings, and there is always a shallowness of affect. In some cases, more severe complications include convulsions and cognitive impairment, and Greenblatt & Myerson (1949) report a mortality rate of between 1 and 4%. Findings such as these, nevertheless, did nothing to dampen enthusiasm for the new technique. For the better part of 20 years – although its limitations were recognised for the treatment of schizophrenia – psychosurgery was used in attempts to treat recurrent depression, obsessional states, severe psychosomatic disorder and intractable pain (Sim 1968).

Electroconvulsive therapy The 1930s also saw the introduction of electroconvulsive therapy (ECT). In this treatment, the person is first given a muscle relaxant and electrodes are fastened to the head. An electric current is applied for less than a second, and the patient throws a convulsion, after which he loses consciousness. On awakening, he is fairly confused and has some degree of memory loss. Following several such treatments, there is generally an alleviation of depressive symptoms; it therefore remains fairly widely used for severe depressions, but not for schizophrenia, where, as with lobotomies, it has not been found to be successful.

Drug therapy In the early part of the century, drugs to treat psychological disorder were available, but their effectiveness was limited. Barbiturates were often used to treat anxiety and insomnia, but they were known to be addictive and to have undesirable side-effects. Reserpine, derived from the plant rauwolfia, is a drug with an even longer history. It was used in India for centuries to treat both physical and mental complaints, and its use spread to the West in the middle of the twentieth century. Principally, the drug was used to treat schizophrenia, but it was also found to have a calming effect on manic elation. In some instances, the side-effects of reserpine are highly undesirable. These include a lowering of blood pressure, limb tremor, swelling of the hands and feet and ineffectiveness in a proportion of cases. It also carries a risk of severe depression in susceptible subjects – an effect which has sometimes led to suicide. In time, the use of reserpine in therapy declined upon the discovery of newer and safer chemical substances.

Antipsychotics. In the 1950s, it was found that a group of drugs, known collectively as the phenothiazines, were effective in treating the symptoms of schizophrenia. Phenothiazine derivatives, such as chlorpromazine, were found to be quick-acting against agitation and thought-disorder; indeed, within a fortnight of treatment, hallucinations are often reduced and may even be eliminated. These 'antipsychotic' drugs block dopamine receptors, thus leading to the theory, already discussed, that excess dopamine is a cause of schizophrenia.

Antidepressants. Following the discovery of the phenothiazines, efforts were made to develop drugs of equal effectiveness for other conditions. In due course, a set of anti-anxiety drugs, known as the minor tranquillisers were developed to reduce tension, and these remain widely used to treat disorders, including depression, in which anxiety is a major feature. Probably the best known of these are Librium and Valium, although each year, many new brands reach the market. However, minor tranquillisers do not help severe depressions. In time, it was discovered that severe cases are best treated by 'energising' chemicals which elevate mood. Today, the two most important antidepressants are the monoamine oxidase (MAO) inhibitors and the tricyclic antidepressants. These appear to operate by increasing the availability of two neurotransmitters, norepinephrine and serotonin.

Advantages of drug therapy. The drugs developed over the past few decades have achieved an objective advocated two hundred years ago by Philippe Pinel (1745–1826). Pinel advocated the removal of chains and iron collars from the mentally ill, and the replacement of such methods by 'moral therapy' and personal attention, with the objective of speeding recovery so that the patient could return to the community and play an active role there. His recommendations were well received, and even implemented in several small 'asylums' but with the introduction and spread of very large psychiatric institutions, it became more and more difficult to implement his policies. An advantage of drug therapy, then, is that people who might formerly have been incarcerated for long periods of their lives can now return home after relatively short periods in hospital. Drug therapy has also put an end to the paraphernalia of previous epochs, including the chains of the eighteenth century, and the straitjackets and padded cells that were to follow.

Achievements of the medical model

The achievements of the medical model are not limited to the development of chemical compounds to treat abnormal behaviour. At the core of the model is the notion that atypical behaviour is symptomatic of an underlying illness. This concept of mental illness has several advantages, a chief one being that it has put paid to previous notions of witchcraft, possession and irresponsibility. Secondly, the notion carries less of a stigma than other explanations since – in theory at least – it is no worse to suffer from a mental illness than from a physical one, such as measles or mumps. Finally, the medical model has inspired a great deal of research into causal factors and possibilities for treatment. Nevertheless, for all this, the model has its critics.

Criticisms of the medical model in psychiatry

Critics of the medical model have challenged the validity of classification systems, and have thus raised questions about diagnostic practices based on these. There are also critics who have cast doubts on the whole concept of mental illness. They argue that, at least in the case of functional disorders, all that is observable is unusual non-conformist behaviour, and that there is no persuasive evidence for an associated illness. At the heart of these criticisms lies the accusation that psychiatric diagnoses involve an unwarranted degree of subjectivity – an ironic charge to level against a system whose original purpose was scientific objectivity.

Unreliability of psychiatric diagnoses

As we have already pointed out, the medical model applies the principles of physical medicine to the diagnosis and treatment of abnormal behaviour. Writing about its original focus, Szasz (1960) observes that the model has clear criteria for distinguishing health from illness because 'the norm is the structural and functional integrity of the human body'. There are, thus, no value judgements inherent in decisions about physical health. However, he notes, subjectivity and value judgements do enter the picture when the physician is diagnosing 'mental illness'. Szasz and other critics further claim that the development of classificatory procedures has not reduced the subjective element in psychiatric diagnoses.

Classifications, past and present, have been attacked on a number of grounds. Attacks include the claim that psychiatric diagnoses are far less reliable than those which pertain to physical medicine, and there is a good deal of evidence to support this claim. Schmidt & Fonda (1956), for example, found that when two psychiatrists used the favoured diagnostic categories of their day, there was a fair agreement on a diagnosis of organic and global psychotic conditions, but a lesser one for subdivisions, including a mere 51% agreement rate for a diagnosis of schizophrenia. Beck (1962) likewise reported only a 54% rate of agreement among four psychiatrists who were asked to diagnose 153 patients within one week of admission to a psychiatric unit. Various attempts have been made to explain away the low diagnostic agreement rates that Beck found, and these would be admissable were it not for the fact that a number of other studies have lent support to his conclusions. The investigation by Schmidt & Fonda backs up Beck's subsequent one, insofar as it pertains to fine diagnostic categories, but other studies suggest that there are difficulties in differentiating even between normal and abnormal behaviour (Box 2.2).

Box 2.2   The Rosenhahn study 1973

The classical study in this field was conducted by Rosenhahn in 1973. While postgraduate practitioners will undoubtedly be acquainted with this, newer practitioners and undergraduates may not be similarly acquainted, and so we shall give a fairly full account of the investigation here. Eight people, including three psychologists, who seemed to be normal by commonsense criteria, went to the admissions office of a mental hospital. Each one complained of hearing noises in his or her head. All were taken into hospital as inpatients, despite the fact that they had not invented any additional symptoms. When questioned on the nature of their noises, they said that they had heard voices saying, 'hollow', 'empty' and 'thud'. That was all they reported. Once they were in hospital, the pseudopatients behaved in a normal fashion. They told staff nurses that they were fine, and spat out any medication administered. The pseudopatients wanted to see how long it would take before they were detected as frauds, but this detection was not forthcoming. Their fellow-patients did suspect that something was amiss – perhaps they were journalists or some other kind of investigator – but the staff diagnosis was one of schizophrenia 'in remission'. They stayed in hospital for an average of 19 days, the range being 7 to 52 days. The implication was that whereas co-patients recognised sanity, medical personnel failed to do so.

Having noted that the diagnostic system of his day could easily describe a 'sane' person as ill, Rosenhahn proceeded to investigate the question of whether an 'ill' person could equally easily be described as 'sane'. Having published the results of his original study, he informed a teaching hospital that within a period of three months, some more pseudopatients would try to gain entry. For the next 193 patients admitted over the experimental period, 41 were alleged to be imposters, and many more were regarded with suspicion, but, in fact, no pseudopatients had presented themselves. This study shows that it is relatively easy to feign mental illness, and that there is a great deal of subjectivity in the diagnoses made by doctors. Following the introduction of DSM-III, it is less likely that misdiagnoses will be made so easily in the future, but this new system has its own problems. For one, it has introduced a label for a whole new host of disordered 'symptoms', and the task of deciding whether these fit a category or not still requires a degree of subjectivity.

Concept of 'mental illness'

The medical model has also been criticised for postulating several 'mental illnesses' which have no known cause. Thus, illness is diagnosed on the basis of presenting symptoms, and the symptoms in turn are said to constitute the illness – a prime example of circular reasoning. Again, the diagnostic criteria are far vaguer in psychiatry than in physical medicine, which uses blood-tests and X-rays to look for signs. For these reasons, Thomas Szasz (1960), a prominent critic of the model, observes that diagnoses always include some kind of value-judgement. He denies that any such entity as 'mental illness' exists, and suggests that in place of the term, we should use the phrase 'problems of living'.

Efficacy of treatment

We have already discussed the procedures used in psychiatry to treat the more severe 'psychotic' disorders, and we have noted that some of the more controversial forms, such as psychosurgical lobotomy, are less frequently used than formerly. Nevertheless, they still have their advocates. Thus, Coleman (1988) quotes from a British Medical Journal of 1984: 'psychosurgery is now clearly indicated in one particular therapeutic situation: that is, when there is a need for 'maintenance' ECT.' Given the nature of these procedures, it is not surprising that the public – not to mention the recipients – look upon them with fear; and there are others who doubt that new drugs really do offer the advantages claimed for them. Mackay (1975), for example, writes that many 'would argue against the "curative" effects of these drugs, and claim that what has happened in the last twenty years is that pharmacological straitjackets have been substituted for those of the more mechanical variety'. Of course, Mackay is right in saying that antipsychotic drugs do not effect a 'cure', since, at least in the case of schizophrenia, discharged persons need to be kept on maintenance doses of phenothiazine drugs. And even when such doses are taken, the rate of relapse is high. As Davison & Neale (1986, p 556) note:

The advent of the 'phenothiazine era' reduced long-term institutionalisation significantly. But in its place evolved the revolving-door pattern of admission, discharge, and readmission already remarked on.

Drug side-effects

A further problem with drug therapy is that its use is by no means limited to the treatment of severe psychiatric disorders, but, as we have seen, is also used to treat a variety of anxiety-related behaviours. Coleman (1988) reports that the prescription of tranquillising drugs derived from benzodiazepine chemicals (e.g. Librium, Valium, Ativan) is on the increase. In 1975, one out of every six British prescriptions was for a drug in this general group. By 1985, roughly three million British people were taking a benzodiazepine drug *every single day*. Early in the 1960s, these drugs were thought to be effective and free from side-effects, certainly by comparison with the barbiturates which preceded them. Nevertheless, over the years, a growing number of side-effects have been highlighted. In the first place, they are highly addictive. Secondly, they are associated with severe depression in some cases, and with memory loss, including retrograde amnesia. Coleman writes that;

many elderly patients had wrongly been diagnosed as senile when in fact it was the drugs they were taking which had affected their ability to think clearly.

(Coleman 1988, p 108)

Coleman offers two reasons for the wholesale prescription of tablets in this way. Firstly, the trend developed once the general public became aware of the link between stress and disease, and began to think that anxiety, irritability and everyday degrees of un-happiness could be treated medically, as diseases. Secondly, Cole-man notes that doctors at that time were not trained to deal with stress-induced problems. Most he says, 'knew little more about anxiety and psychosomatic disease than their patients. Indeed many probably knew far less'. Yet for all that has since become known about both stress and the side-effects of popular tranquillisers, 'and despite the fact that they are more addictive than heroin, these drugs are still prescribed by the lorryload'.

'Radical' psychiatry

The views of R D Laing

Together with Thomas Szasz, Ronald Laing is probably the best-known critic of the medical model. It is of interest that both are medical doctors, specialising in psychiatry. Laing's special concern is schizophrenia which, like Szasz, he believes is not a mental illness but, rather, a particular way of experiencing the world. His position is an existentialist-phenomenological one which advocates concern for the client's subjective views over 'symptoms' diagnosed by the observer. However, for convenience and to aid communication, he continues to use the terms 'schizophrenia' and 'patient'. The seeds of Laing's viewpoint were sown early during his training in Glas-gow. In a retrospective account of his early doubts about labelling, Laing (1976) recalled a case conference during the 1950s in which the patient under consideration was a young man with a feeling of futility. Staff were pondering whether his case should be diagnosed as one of schizoid personality or schizophrenia itself in its early stages. Laing noted that he intervened:

to remark that the question whether life was worth living had been taken up quite a bit in recent European literature, indeed one could find considerations of it all over the place. I did not think it a foregone conclusion that the sense of futility betokened psychopathology.

(Laing 1976, p 110)

In Laing's first book, *The Divided Self* (1960), he argued that many so-called symptoms were perfectly understandable reactions to certain kinds of stress.

Laing's account of schizophrenia is that it is a strategy developed by an 'ontologically insecure' individual to deal with some intolerable situation. Being insecure, the person is terrified of events and relationships that might destroy his identity. The person's experience is that he has two selves: one is the physical self – really a 'false' self, presented to society – and the other a detached and private 'inner' self. Under pressure, the false self alone communicates with other people, while the individual otherwise retreats from reality into his inner world where he feels safer amid his delusions and hallucinations. Laing (1964) describes the intolerable position of the schizophrenic as one in which he is bombarded by contradictory pressures which cannot be escaped. He is caught in a 'double-bind' trap, since even if he does nothing at all he will still merit censure. In his later writings, Laing indicated that, in some situations, family influences were at the root of schizophrenic reactions. However, as Browne (1990) points out, he was not critical of the family per se, merely observing that there are bad as well as good family influences.

Laing's view of treatment is that it should, above all, recognise the validity and meaning of the person's experience, and use this recognition to try and heal the characteristic split. His perception of schizophrenia is that it is not qualitatively different from 'normal' experience, and he holds that the therapist must acknowledge this if he is to help the patient on his 'voyage' of discovery. If he does not, and if he chooses to focus only on the removal of symptoms, all that can be achieved is a temporary rehabilitation of the false self. In the 1960s, Laing set up his own therapeutic community at Kingsley Hall in London. Here, in line with existentialist principles, community members shared in the experience of each individual, giving support where necessary to those who wished to make regressive journeys back through the traumas of childhood. It has been said of Laing that he selected for therapy only those who had a good 'prognosis', and there are others who complain that it is impossible to replicate his procedures since he did not use objective measures, controls and statistics. While there appears to be some truth in the first accusation, it is unrealistic to expect of Laing that he conform to the detached and objective attitude of science. The whole point of his argument is that it is this very attitude that dehumanises the person and reduces his status to that of a 'thing'.

As an existentialist, Laing places a high value on personal freedom and authenticity. He argues that the person's authenticity is denied when he is viewed objectively by the interviewer only in terms of symptoms; moreover, the hospital routine can add to this sense of depersonalisation. He argues further that the individual's right to freedom is eroded when he is admitted to hospital against his will, and subjected to treatments about which he is not consulted.

Influence of 'radical' psychiatry

The views of Laing, Szasz and other 'radical' psychiatrists have had an enormous impact on research. Over the past two decades, investigators have turned again to a study of family relationships in schizophrenia, and many pathologies of communication have been found (Fontana 1966, Lidz 1973, Norton 1982). However, it is by no means clear that these play a causal role. They may be responses to the problem of having a schizophrenic child in the family, or they may indeed be predictors as Goldstein & Rodnick (1975) found in a follow-up study of adolescents. Goldstein later reported (1985) that schizophrenia is more likely to occur in a context of confused communication patterns *combined* with negative and rejecting parental attitudes. Currently, several longitudinal studies of 'high-risk' children are in progress which, in due course, will further our understanding of the contributory factors. It has also been found that family atmosphere has an impact on relapse rates. Where parents and spouses are overtly critical, hostile, or over-involved emotionally, discharged schizophrenics are over five times more likely to relapse than are patients who return to homes with low 'expressed emotion' (Leff 1976).

As the so-called radical 'anti-psychiatry' movement gained ground, the media brought its claims to public attention. Films such as *Family Life* and *One Flew Over the Cuckoo's Nest* pleaded the case for an alternative view of mental illness and more humane forms of treatment. In time, governments took note. Many countries, including Britain, followed Italy's lead and began to close down large institutions, especially the older, Victorian-style asylums. In Britain, the reforms of the 1983 Mental Health Act were designed to copper-fasten the individual's right to freedom, and it became ever more difficult to detain people compulsorily.

Finally, doctors grew reluctant to admit patients to hospital unless it was vital and, wherever possible, outpatient treatment and community care was advocated. But has the pendulum swung too far, and are communities sufficiently equipped to offer the provisions now demanded of them? Debate on these issues continues during the 1990s, and present trends will be discussed in the final chapter of this book.

THE SCOPE OF THE MEDICAL MODEL

In their book, 'Follies and Fallacies in Medicine', Skrabanek & McCormick (1989) have drawn attention to flaws in logic that characterise thinking in the field. The authors are medical doctors and university lecturers, and place a high value on critical appraisal, acknowledging (p 1) that progress in science depends 'upon clearing away rubbish and challenging accepted dogma and belief'. Among the fallacies discussed are those which assume that association implies causality, those which hold that authority is necessarily right, and those which pertain to diagnostic error ('When in doubt, diagnose.'). Above all, the authors highlight 'the fallacy that an alteration in symptoms following treatment is necessarily a specific result of that therapy' (p 3), and they point out that placebo effects and the healing power of nature are too often overlooked.

Thinking simplistically about intervention is most likely to occur in the context of a circumscribed model, and, of course, the medical approach is reductionist in that explanations and attempts to cure focus principally on physicochemical aspects of the person. This is not to say that all doctors take a reductionist view of the human beings they care for. There are exceptions, and some doctors do attempt to grapple with the psychological and social problems of their patients. Nevertheless, the medical model inclines practitioners to reductionism, so that despite the frequent doubts that have been aired, the prescription of chemical and physical remedies continues prolifically.

The authors do not take the view, held by Illich, that improvements in health today have little or nothing to do with medicine. The role of medicine in preventing disease by innoculation, in treating disease itself, and in offering surgery to relieve pain and prevent death is fully acknowledged. Nevertheless, it must be said that the effectiveness of medicine is limited to well-defined disease entities and deficiencies, and that this is so because its theories are constrained by the core of the medical model which is oriented to physical causes and physico-chemical forms of treatment. Several examples have been provided of how the model has been extended far beyond its range of application, and that there exists a degree of doubt about its influence on psychiatry has been indicated. Thus, Coleman (1988) writes that: 'Twentieth-century psychiatry is more of a black art than a science', and MacKay (1975, p 130) concludes that:

Perhaps the most serious charge levied against the medical model is that it has ceased to develop. The only new research findings these days are those concerned with new psychotropic drugs which purport to eliminate symptoms more effectively, and give rise to fewer side effects, than their predecessors.'

We have observed that the medical model is most flawed where it overextends its scope. Given this, there is emphatically a need – logically and psychologically – for alternative, holistic approaches. When occupational therapy is compared with medicine, however, it is too often deemed inferior because it has a lesser range, although its own areas of competence remain acknowledged. The question that must be asked, then, is whether medicine's scope is in fact as wide as its protagonists claim. The authors are persuaded by the arguments and evidence which suggest that it is not. It would appear that medical treatment is effective in *some* circumstances, but not in all. This is also the claim that is generally made for occupational therapy.

Scientific concepts and professional development

This chapter has tried to demonstrate that medical science is no different from any other form of science. It is founded on a set of basic hypotheses or theories, some of whose deductions have led to effective forms of treatment, and some of which have not. In general, medicine advances by adhering to a set of basic assumptions which guide research. These pertain to the physical basis of disease, and have been maintained even when hypotheses derived from them have been refuted. It has been suggested, for example by Mocellin (1984), that occupational therapy should proceed along similar lines.

Mocellin

Mocellin (1984) notes that, for a time, most occupational therapists followed Kielhofner & Burke's (1982) use of the term, 'paradigm', to account for professional development, until its connotations of irrationality and dogmatism were recognised. Given this limitation, Mocellin suggests that we use instead 'a modified version of Lakatos' concept of scientific research programmes'. His modification proposes that the hard core defines the profession's characteristics:

It takes the form of some very general theoretical concepts that form the basis from which the profession develops. The hard-core is never changed and any therapist who modifies the hard-core would no longer be called an occupational therapist.

(Mocellin 1984, p 11)

The protective belt, on the other hand, is 'that aspect of the profession which indicates the kind of things occupational therapists should do. It should offer to the profession opportunity for new discoveries and a chance to realize its full potential'.

Mocellin quotes with approval several writers who have suggested that occupational therapy should move away from the medical-reductionist model. Yet, having voiced agreement with them, he proceeds to compare medicine and occupational therapy, using the modified Lakatos model, and finds that occupational therapy compares very unfavourably. Relative to medicine, he claims, its hard core is ill-defined and unprotected. Medicine's protective belt has a specific focus, it is specialised and scientific, while that of occupational therapy is shared with many others, often promotes aimless development and frequently is seen as the hard core. Medical intervention is specific and often 'dramatic and visible'; occupational therapy intervention is general and its results hard to quantify. Mocellin further submits that there is currently considerable professional ambivalence among occupational therapists who, apparently, 'do not know what to do'.

An important point to make about Mocellin's picture of medicine as a model science is that much of its success in this sphere is due to the very fact that it is reductionist. Thus, just as some branches of psychology early this century postulated little difference between rat and human behaviour, and so could develop simple testable hypotheses, medical hypotheses are likewise relatively easy to test wherever health problems are reduced to categories of disease. However, we cannot generalise from the rat to the human, nor can we assume that all instances of ill-health should be treated purely as physical defects or diseases. It is this central assumption of the medical model that has most frequently been attacked. It is worth noting, too, that if occupational therapists are currently ambivalent about their profession, so too are many physicians about theirs. Indeed, the majority of critics we have quoted are themselves medical practitioners.

While acknowledging the achievements and recent advances of medicine, Skrabanek & McCormick (1989) have chosen to review their own discipline in a sceptical light. To do so, they point out, is not to suggest that medicine is a threat to health:

Medicine only becomes a threat to health if it remains untempered by the use of rational inquiry and criticism. Such criticism is an important and relatively neglected task.

(Skrabanek & McCormick 1989, p 143)

And the authors conclude (p 144):

Scepticism is the scalpel which frees accessible truth from the dead tissue of unfounded belief and wishful thinking. The demarcation of ignorance and the exposure of folly may diminish harm, and by removing some of the rubble which impedes the way forward, accelerate progress.

Critical self-examination can benefit professional development. In the case of occupational therapy, there is a need to eschew defensiveness in the face of criticism and accept its advantages. There is a need, too, to review the considerable body of theory that underpins our profession and develop criteria for selecting those principles that best represent its core. But there are constraints on this process. Occupational therapy cannot be based on a mechanistic 'closed system' view of human beings (Kielhofner 1985). Its core must comprise theories that are compatible with a holistic, humanistic perspective.

3. Frames of reference in occupational therapy

PHILOSOPHICAL INFLUENCES

The philosophical antecedents of occupational therapy can be traced back through the cultures of ancient China, Persia, Greece and Egypt. A comprehensive overview of these roots may be found in the excellent accounts of Licht (1978), Hopkins (1982) and MacDonald (1978).

During the eighteenth and nineteenth centuries, in both Europe and the United States, there began an upsurge of concern for persons incarcerated as lunatics. This concern was partly the outcome of humanistic perceptions of Quakers, and partly the result of the political upheaval generated by the revolutions in France and the United States. This new perception of the insane was known as 'moral treatment', and sought to replace physical restraint with diversions and work to prevent the effects of idleness and boredom. Possibly the first publication concerned with occupational therapy was by a Frenchman, Leuret (1840) writing on the moral treatment of insanity. More recently, J. Sanbourne Buckoven (1971) urged occupational therapists to reclaim their roots in moral treatment, and suggested that the value of occupational therapy lies in its respect for the realities of life, for the real task of living and for the time it takes the individual to develop his modes of coping with his tasks. It is this commitment which should encourage occupational therapy to go its own way (away from medicine) to fulfil its professional destiny.

The Hungarian, Alfred Korzybski, who lived in the United States, and was the founder of the 'Non-Aristotelian Society', spent much time considering the nature and purpose of humanity. His writings reflected on classes of life: plants, he wrote: (Korzybski 1921), are 'chemistry-bound', that is, they remain static and depend for life on chemical substances, either in the soil or brought to them; animals are 'space-bound', that is they may move from place to place in order to meet their needs; and humanity is 'time-bound'. Not only may mankind move freely to meet his needs, but he is also able to know about and inspect his past, and plan for his future; he may also use his understanding of the past to attempt to alter his present and thus his predictable future.

It was in part this concept of humanity as a time-bound class of life that influenced the thinking of Adolph Meyer, an eminent American psychiatrist who saw that one value of 'occupation' was that it structured time between birth and death, that occupation may be inspected and therefore altered. He wrote that 'the proper use of time in some helpful and justifying activity appeared to be a fundamental issue in the treatment of the patient' (Meyer 1922). More recently, the medical philosopher, H. Tristram Engelhardt (1977) suggested that the unique contribution of occupational therapy was through its stress on fulfilment through human activity. Engelhardt (1974) defined health care as 'helping human organisms to do things. Humans are healthy or diseased in terms of the activities and functions open to them or denied them.'

The Australian occupational therapist, George Mocellin (1984), suggests that it is indeed the experience of doing – of efficacy, of control and of self-determination – that is therapeutic, not the occupation itself. He defines the experience as 'competency', a term taken by White (1971) to mean sufficiency or adequacy to meet the demands of a situation or task. Mocellin reflects that competency does not equate with excellence, normality or the ability to do everything, and that norms for competence vary with age, culture, personal abilities and values. Functional competence may thus be age-graded, socially defined and individually specific.

Historically, then, thinking about occupational therapy began as a practical implementation of moral treatment. It became associated with ideas about humanity's use of time, and a perception of health as the ability to function, and now defines this functioning in terms of competent behaviour. To take this process further, it is suggested that it is competent behaviour in the occupations related to productivity, leisure and self-care, in balance and combination, that engages the attention and endeavours of humankind between life and death. It is an interest in such competency that provides the philosophical perspective of our profession.

Translating philosophy into theory

Since the 1980s, serious attempts have been made by occupational therapists to translate the philosophy of occupational therapy into theories whose assumptions may be tested and which may be used to develop frames of reference for a unique practice. This has proved a complex task, not least because of the diversity of existing practice and the wide range of clients with whom we seek to intervene. It is, however, a worthwhile task, as the lack of tested theories and of clearly defined frames of reference results in professional fragmentation and leaves unanswered the question 'What is occupational therapy?' One early attempt was made by Reed (1984) who reviewed existing 'models for practice', and offered an analysis of the construction of a 'practice model'. However, the all-embracing 'model for practice' still eludes us. Perhaps this is not surprising. Mosey (1989) indicates that such a model would need to include 'all of a profession's beliefs, philosophical assumptions and knowledge' – a tall order, to say the least, and one that may not be desirable. After all, a model, although useful, is a means for making the abstract concrete, and cannot substitute for testable theories.

Kuhn

Kuhn's notion of a 'paradigm' was then put forward. Kuhn had suggested that scientific enquiry proceeds by discarding out-moded theories when, after a period of uncertainty and confusion, they are replaced by a new, more acceptable theory, thus making progress towards an ever clearer understanding of the science being studied. This notion was attractive to occupational therapy; our practice had, indeed, moved forward as new knowledge became available, and it was tempting to describe new advances as a move from paradigm to paradigm. However, for occupational therapists to embrace this notion poses difficulties. Occupational therapy is an applied science, and the knowledge base for our practice is derived, in large measure, from the basic sciences; for us to use *Their* new knowledge to develop *Our* new paradigms circumvents the requirement for occupational therapy to generate and test its own theories. Futhermore, repeated periods of uncertainty, between paradigms, produces a lack of stability in practice. However, the greatest disadvantage of the 'paradigm' notion is the revelatory nature of a new paradigm,and the perception that it is virtually unchallengeable.

Lakatos

Lakatos suggested that some measure of stability may be main-

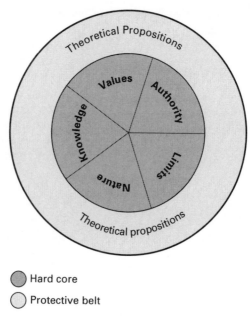

Fig. 3.1 Occupational therapy as a hard core of knowledge with a protective belt of theories.

tained through theory change by the identification of a *hard core* of knowledge which is surrounded and protected by a *belt* of theoretical propositions (Fig. 3.1), all of which are subjected to increasingly rigorous testing in an endeavour to falsify them. Until they are falsified they are retained, and may be extended by additional hypotheses. This repeated and rigorous testing is to be encouraged, provided the modus tollens (or falsification principle) is aimed away from the hard core.

The present authors support Lakatos' suggestions as the most useful in the continuing search for a scientific base for the practice of occupational therapy, for the following reasons:

- a stable hard core prevents confusion and instability
- the search for one unifying model for practice may be a long time coming, even if desirable
- we need different frames of reference, not only, as Clark (1979) suggests, because of the diverse nature of our practice, but also because they are derived from theories which have not been thoroughly tested, and it thus seems premature to discard them.

An attempt will now be made to use the structure suggested by Lakatos for a programme of research applicable to occupational therapy. A hard core will be proposed and it will be suggested that there exist theories for a protective belt. That our practice may be specific when derived from theoretically sound frames of reference will be indicated. In doing so, it is hoped to meet the challenge of Mocellin (1984), contained in his statement that the hard core of occupational therapy is 'very small, ill defined . . . [and has] . . . little professional allegiance'. The authors do not dispute this indictment, but suggest that the hard core and protective belt do exist, although they have not previously been identified.

THE HARD CORE

The authors propose that the hard core of occupational therapy comprises five elements (Fig. 3.1):

1. the *Values* of practice
2. the *Authority* for practice
3. the *Knowledge* for practice
4. the *Nature* of practice
5. the *Limits* of practice.

Each of these elements will now be examined in some detail.

Values of practice

In a presentation to occupational therapists in the United States Engelhardt (1986) reminded us that it is the values of a profession that must be the touchstone of practice. Our professional values have been codified by Yerxa (1980; Box 3.1).
Accepting these values as the touchstone of practice, we seek the active involvement of our clients to become participants in improving their own performance. We see them as actively influencing their environment in order to maintain or enhance their own health.

Authority for practice

Siegler & Osmond (1974) suggest that the authority for medical practice derives from the patient's fear of death, and that the Greco-Roman god of medicine, called Aesculapius, gives physicians Aesculapian authority to practise medicine. This authority encompasses three kinds of power:

Box 3.1   Professional values as codified by Yerxa (1980)

1. We value the essential humanity of the client and acknowledge an obligation for life satisfaction of the severely disabled.
2. We value the maintenance and enhancement of health.
3. We value the self-directedness and responsibility of the client.
4. We value a generalist, integrated view of the client.
5. We value a therapeutic relationship of mutual cooperation with the client.
6. We value the client acting on their environment rather than being determined by it.
7. We have faith in the potential of the client.
8. We acknowledge that the client is productive and participates in treatment.
9. We acknowledge that play and leisure activities are essential components of a balanced life.
10. We acknowledge the subjective perspective of the client.

- the right to control and direct patients based on moral authority – the goodness of the medical ethic
- the right to control and direct patients based on charismatic authority – a God-given grace as a healer of diseases
- the right to give advice and to be heard by reason of knowledge and expertise – based on sapiential authority.

Yerxa (1980) expounds on this theme in two articles, and suggests that it is only this sapiential authority which we, as a profession, may justly claim – we have no moral authority to control or direct our patients, nor do we have a God-given charismatic authority. We can, however, claim the right to give advice and to be heard by reason of our knowledge and expertise. Sapiential authority does not conflict with our values, which clearly indicate our recognition of patients' rights to control their own lives.

Knowledge for practice

The clients with whom we intervene are dysfunctional. This dysfunction is usually the outcome of some kind of pathology –

biological, psychosocial or the outcome of a hostile social context. In order for us to understand the impact of pathology, we must be well versed in the basic sciences – the biological, behavioural and medical sciences. We are also concerned with human beings throughout their lifespan, and with the uniqueness of each individual. We therefore need a knowledge of normal human development in all its various aspects, and at all ages 'from cradle to grave'. Our intervention strategies focus on the occupations and activities appropriate and acceptable within their social context. Thus, the third essential knowledge base must focus on an understanding of activity and its role in inducing health and restoring the human organism.

The knowledge for practice comes from the basic sciences, from an understanding of human development and from the role of activity in competent human functioning. It should, however, be noted that all the so-called 'helping professions' – educators, probation officers, as well as all the medical and health-related professions – claim their knowledge from some aspect of human development and that an understanding of human development derives from the basic sciences. Thus, we can hardly claim that this knowledge base is unique to occupational therapy. As we strive towards fully-fledged professional status and identifying as ours a unique body of knowledge, we must, therefore, look to the third area of knowledge from which our practice comes – that of *activity*.

The central role of activity in our practice was recognised by the AOTA representative assembly (1979) in a statement which includes the sentence, 'Activity as used by the occupational therapist includes both an intrinsic and a therapeutic purpose'. The European Committee on Occupational Therapy (1989) agreed on the definition quoted in Chapter 1 as follows: 'Occupational therapists assess and treat people using purposeful activity to prevent disability, and develop independent function.'[†] The central role of activity in the practice of occupational therapy is discussed in detail in Chapters 6 and 7.

Nature of practice

In keeping with our values, and based on sapiential authority; equipped with our knowledge, derived from the basic sciences, of activity and human development, how do occupational therapists

---

[†] COTEC (1989)

intervene? What is the nature of our practice? There have been several suggestions as to the outcome of occupational therapy intervention. Kielhofner suggests that occupational therapists intervene 'by replacing the lost occupation with carefully graded and organised activities'. Reed indicates that occupational therapists intervene 'to prevent, restore or maintain skills and functions'. Rather fewer suggestions have been offered as to *how* any of this is to occur. West (1984) indicates that education has always been a major tool in occupational therapy intervention and Mocellin (1984) takes this idea further by suggesting that occupational therapists teach their clients 'all manner of skills'. These ideas, however, do not seem to satisfy the stated values of our profession, in which we perceive our clients as active on their own behalf, and the role of the occupational therapist as cooperative, rather than directive or prescriptive.

Perhaps it would be helpful to back-track a little and suggest that the hoped-for outcome of intervention is a change in the behaviour of our client which will provide an incremental step in reaching the client's own identified goal; such a change may be to do with self-care, productivity or leisure, and thus with the client's active influence on his or her own environment. Change may occur in three ways (Fig. 3.2).

- chemical change when the physiology of the body is changed through the ingestion or injection of chemical substance
- mechanical change when the anatomy of the body is changed,

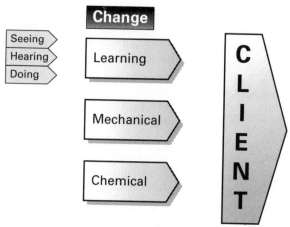

Fig. 3.2 Ways in which change can occur in the client.

often by surgery followed by the addition of a man-made substitute, like an artificial limb or dentures
- change through learning, which has been defined by Craig (1976) as 'that which produces a relatively permanent change in behaviour or in the capacity for behaviour, resulting from either experience or practice.'

We know that the process of learning takes place through the senses, through seeing, hearing and doing. The nature of our practice, then, may be stated as providing opportunities for our clients to learn, using their own senses, in order to produce a change in their behaviour which will more usefully influence their own environment. Reilly (1962) more eloquently reflected that 'man, through the use of his hands as they are energised by mind and will, can influence the state of his own health'.

Limits of practice

Our practice must be limited by our values; limited to that which requires the participation of our clients in improving their own performance in order actively to influence their own environment as they themselves dictate. Our practice must be limited by our authority: the authority to give advice and be heard by reason of our knowledge. Our practice must be limited by our knowledge: our knowledge of the basic sciences, of human development and, above all, our knowledge of the role of activity in promoting competent human performance. Our practice must be limited by its own nature: limited to providing opportunities for our clients to learn so that change may take place.

Only by imposing these limits on our practice may we identify the uniqueness of occupational therapy, and so begin to satisfy our hope of becoming a fully-fledged profession.

THE PROTECTIVE BELT

Having proposed a hard core specific to occupational therapy, we shall now continue with the model suggested by Lakatos, and proceed to identify some existing theoretical frames of reference which will serve to protect and harden this core. Much of the theoretical knowledge from which occupational therapy practice is derived is shared with other professions; it is our frames of reference which specify the nature, aims and procedures that distinguish the appli-

Box 3.2   Frames of reference

1. Adaptive performance
   Proposed by Fidler and Mosey from a theoretical base
   in psychiatry or psychoanalysis, notably the work of
   Freud, Jung and Sullivan.
2. Developmental
   Proposed by Llorens, Ayres and Arieti from the
   theories of Piaget, Freud and Erikson.
3. Sensorimotor
   Proposed by de Quiros and Ayres from a theoretical
   base in the neurosciences.
4. Cognitive
   Proposed by Allen from a theoretical base in the
   neurosciences and activity analysis.
5. Role performance
   Proposed by Reilly, Kielhofner and Shannon from a
   theoretical base in general systems theory development,
   notably the work of Boulding, von Bertolanffy and
   Brunner.
6. Rehabilitation
   Proposed by Spackman and Tromley from a theoretical
   base in the physical sciences.

cation of theory for occupational therapists from the application
used by others. Clark (1979) discusses four frames of reference;
Hopkins (1988) identifies nine of them. The present authors plan
to be selective and we shall discuss firstly those frames of reference
which are most protective of the hard core. Six such frames of reference are proposed (Box 3.2) and a brief review of each is offered.
The extent to which they provide a 'belt' to both protect and
harden the core of occupational therapy will then be discussed.

Adaptive performance

Fidler and Mosey are the occupational therapists who have developed theoretical constructs which suggest that the performance of
the client who is engaged on some concrete task is an area of interest to the occupational therapist. The concrete, enduring nature
of the completed task permits inspection by clients of the outcome
of their own performance, and thus offers a means by which the
client may identify behaviour to be changed. For example, a client

engaged in some simple task, such as setting type for the wording on a greeting card, may himself see that his insistence on doing this task again and again until it is 'perfect' will inhibit progress and impede performance. Clients are thus provided with an opportunity to identify behaviour in need of change. Furthermore, occupational therapy may then provide a safe setting within which the client may experiment by learning ways in which to change this behaviour – the role of the occupational therapist being to provide these opportunities for learning.

Fidler extends this notion to suggest the possibility of a similar experience in which, when working in groups, clients may also identify inhibiting behaviour in their own interpersonal skills. By working with others on some concrete project, they may come to recognise that their behaviour in ignoring the needs of other group members to use tools, to express creativity or to give and receive encouragement may inhibit productivity and impair relationships. The occupational therapist enables the client to identify behaviour in need of change, and then to learn and experiment with ways in which change may occur.

In 1968, Mosey expanded this thinking about the practice of occupational therapy to include that which she termed the 're-capitulation of ontogenesis'. Not only, she suggests, may the client identify and seek to change maladaptive performance behaviour, but he also has a chance to 'recapitulate – to go back and re-solve the problems of psychosocial development. For example, using Erikson's framework for the stages of this aspect of development, a client who, for whatever reasons, had previously learned to operate from a stance of 'shame' is enabled to go back, have another chance, and learn the alternative stance of 'autonomy'. Here again, the role of the occupational therapist is that of providing opportunities for learning.

Developmental

Llorens postulates that as human development may be inspected both vertically and horizontally, so intervention may occur to facilitate this process at any stage and in any area. In other words, for each individual, normal growth and development proceeds predictably, sequentially and cumulatively in terms of sensorimotor, psychosocial, language and cognitive development. Each stage of development is more or less age-related, so may also be inspected across the spectrum of development; it may then be seen that at any given age a normally developing individual will have attained skills in all areas of development. For example, by the age of about two years, a normally developing child is able to use a spoon and fork, manage large buttons and turn taps on and off; she is also using language to communicate and is beginning to establish some sort of psychological independence; thus development has a horizontal nature. However, each of the areas of development also occurs vertically, building on previously acquired skills and making possible progress in the developmental process. Llorens suggests that interference in any aspect of development will influence development in *all* areas. She also suggests that carefully selected, specific activity may be used to facilitate or remediate developmental insufficiencies. In order to 'carefully select' the most appropriate activity to promote facilitation, both the client's performance and possible remedial activities must be analysed.

In a paper published in 1989, Llorens demonstrates such an analysis. This particular theoretical framework requires the therapist to evaluate the client's present performance, which may lead to a prescriptive mode of intervention. Although the remediation process seeks the active participation of the client in 'doing', and thereby learning in order to promote change, it also relies on the knowledge of the therapist in terms of development and of activity, and on the skill of the therapist in providing specific learning opportunities, and so remains within the suggested limits of occupational therapy practice. One notable feature is that the therapist is required to be expert in analysing activity, both the activities currently being performed by the client and those selected as most likely to facilitate change. The whole issue of activity analysis is central to this and other theories for the practice of occupational therapy, and Chapter 7 is devoted to this subject.

Sensorimotor

Ayres and Wilbarger are the two individuals most generally associated with theories related to *sensory integration*. They suggest that occupational therapy is the science of eliciting an adaptive response, and that the sensory-integrative process facilitates an appropriate response to incoming information. Maladaptive responses may produce anxiety, disruptive behaviour and inadequate intellectual performance. Most work, to date, has focused on the vestibular and tactile systems, and is firmly grounded in a knowledge of the neurosciences, Piaget's suggestions regarding cognition (Box 4.1) and the study of physiological psychology. Ayres indicates that clients frequently identify their own needs, although much of the intervention offered is premised on the therapist's knowledge of human development and activity, and the very exact use and interpretation of precise evaluation instruments. The client learns in order to promote change, although the means for learning includes special equipment, the use and proper application of which requires skill on the part of the therapist.

Cognitive

In 1985, Claudia Allen published a book with the stated purpose of identifying the nature and severity of cognitive disabilities which accompany a wide spectrum of mental diseases (Allen 1985). She then focused on the client population with whom most occupational therapists practise, namely the chronically impaired. She suggested that as diminished cognitive ability in this group is likely to be permanent, the role of the occupational therapist could be that of measuring the residual cognitive function and then of contributing to the management of clients as they try to function in a community, as opposed to an institutional, environment. The knowledge needed to implement Allen's suggestions is derived from the basic sciences and from a thorough understanding of activity, the analysis of activity as well as its use in measuring cognitive function. Allen identified six levels of cognitive function, level 1 being the most restricted, and limited to the performance of automatic actions like eating, drinking and walking, while level 6 is the least restricted and includes the capacity to plan ahead. Allen also developed and offers the Allen Cognitive Level Test for the assessment of cognitive performance.

Role performance

The occupational behaviour of human beings forms the focus of frames of reference for the practice of occupational therapy initially developed by Reilly. Her work has been extended by a cohort of others, each of whom contributed to this theoretical construct which has come to preoccupy many occupational therapists, initially in the United States and, more recently, in Canada, Australia, the United Kingdom and Ireland. Reilly initially postulated that the 'occupation' of human beings could be classified as 'work, play, rest and sleep'. She and her associates undertook extensive study and research in the areas of work and play, with the result that they have developed a considerable body of knowledge relative to the functions, tasks, habits and skills required to fulfil occupational roles. Matsutsuyu suggested that occupational behaviour must be seen in a sociological context of 'role'; and Heard extended these ideas to work with the chronically sick. As ideas related to occupational behaviour and role fulfilment have developed, they have become allied both with the philosophical notions of general system theory, which sees mankind as the creator of his own world, and also, more recently with Kuhn's notion of 'paradigm', which offers a rationale for regarding 'occupational behaviour' as an all-embracing theoretical construct for the practice of occupational therapy. Kielhofner and Barris have written extensively on the relationship between this theoretical construct and the practice of occupational therapy, and have developed assessment tools and goals for intervention.

To date, the construction of this theoretical framework remains more of an art than a science, although some serious efforts have been made to collect and inspect hard scientific data to support the theories. Essentially, clients do identify their own needs, although often through interview rather than through the use of concrete activity; the knowledge required of the therapist is based on the 'role' outcomes of human development, and the skills of the therapist include an extensive grasp of activity. The nature of occupational therapy intervention relevant to this theoretical framework is unclear, although presumably clients learn skills either to replace or to extend those needed for more adequate role performance. This particular frame of reference is certainly promising, the present authors are hopeful that the emerging theory will not be extended so far or so fast that the scientific underpinning is hard-pushed to support the notions embodied in it.

Rehabilitation

Rehabilitation, including amputation and prosthetics, self-care, architectural barriers and pre-vocational evaluation, seeks to find compensatory ways for clients to function, in a way acceptable to them, when they need to live with a disability on a temporary or permanent basis. It focuses on seeking ways in which the client may attain an optimal level of independence; this can include the use of special equipment, which is often available commercially or, in rare instances, is fabricated by the therapist. Evaluation is specific to the needs of the individual client, and is frequently accomplished through the use of check lists. Treatment techniques are specific and focused on meeting the needs of the individual client. Clients are encouraged to identify their own needs. The therapist's contribution stems from her understanding of the effects of trauma on human functioning, and of the therapeutic use of activities. Clients learn through activity to promote change, which may be to do with alternative ways of functioning, or with the outcome of environmental change, particularly when disability is permanent. The practice of occupational therapy focused on rehabilitation does, therefore, seem to support the hard care of occupational therapy practice.

REVIEW

Each of the six frames of reference for the practice of occupational therapy discussed above recognises the ability of the client to be self-directed, productive and responsible, and to act on his environment rather than be determined by it. Each frame of reference requires a collaborative endeavour between client and therapist, who offers advice which stems from our knowledge, is in accord with our values and stays within the bounds of our authority. Each is based on the legitimate knowledge of occupational therapists, and each relies on the client's learning in order to promote change, so staying within the limits suggested for practice. These frames of reference are, however, just that; most are stronger in their 'art' form – as notions about occupational therapy – than they are as science. They tend to lack hypotheses which may be falsified. However, were we, as a profession, to focus our attention on developing a real programme of research designed to develop and test hypotheses from these frames of reference, we may well produce valuable theories, unique to occupational therapy, theories which would continue to protect and harden the core of our practice.

There is one characteristic shared by the frames of reference here reviewed. Although each was proposed as applicable to a specific client population, each holds the potential for use with all the clients we traditionally treat. The ideas inherent in 'adaptive performance' could be as useful to the physically impaired as to the psychiatric clients for whom they were developed. Llorens' suggestions based on developmental theory are clearly applicable 'across the board', so too are those inherent in the sensorimotor, cognitive and role performance frames of reference. The rehabilitation of the psychiatric client is already addressed by occupational therapists;

the implementation strategies differ from those useful with the physically impaired, but the essential concepts remain the same.

Maybe, just maybe, if we are able to generate theories of our own from these frames of reference, we will be able to proceed to the building of that much sought after, but so far elusive, model for practice in occupational therapy.

The reader may well have noticed the omission of three frames of reference often included in overviews of occupational therapy

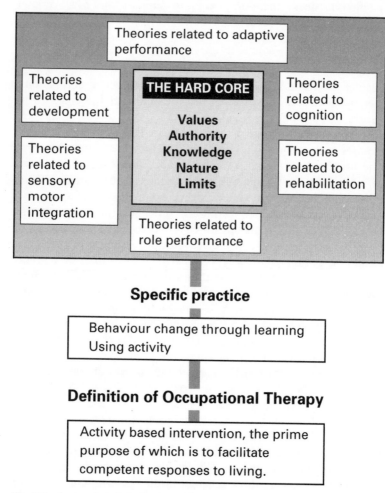

Specific practice

Behaviour change through learning
Using activity

Definition of Occupational Therapy

Activity based intervention, the prime
purpose of which is to facilitate
competent responses to living.

Fig. 3.3 A representation of concepts derived from the model proposed by Lakatos and applied to occupational therapy.

practice – the biomechanical, proposed by Tromley; the neuro-developmental, proposed by Bobath and Rood, among others; and the behavioural, based on the work of Skinner. The authors do not question for a moment that practice based on these frames of reference may be of great and real benefit to selected clients. However, they tend to be prescriptive in nature and to stem from an Aesculapian rather than a sapiential authority – to be more compatible with a medical model for practice than with a model aspired to by occupational therapy. For these reasons they have not been included in this particular review.

That the frames of reference for occupational therapy we have reviewed originate in the United States is not surprising as, for a number of years, occupational therapists in that country have been engaged in graduate level research. As, throughout Europe and elsewhere, an increasing number of occupational therapists have the same opportunities, professional research programmes will develop on this side of the Atlantic.

In summary, this chapter has sought, through a modification of Lakatos' ideas about scientific research, to identify the 'hard core' of occupational therapy practice. Six existing frames of reference used to support practice were then inspected, in an endeavour to see whether or to what extent these theories provide a protective belt for the hard core. It is now suggested that practice *is* specific, and focuses on promoting change through client-learning by the use of activity. We also suggest that the practice of occupational therapy may be defined as 'activity-based intervention, the prime purpose of which is to facilitate competent responses to living'.

Figure 3.3 presents in diagrammatic form the hard core, the protective belt, the specificity of practice and a definition of occupational therapy.

4. Concepts of occupational therapy: understanding development

THE CONCEPT OF DEVELOPMENT

In Chapter 3, it was suggested that knowledge for the practice of occupational therapy is drawn from three sources – from the basic sciences, from theories of human development, and from an understanding of activity and its role in both promoting and restoring competent function. There are numerous textbooks devoted to the basic sciences. In this book, therefore, we shall concentrate on human development as a knowledge base of occupational therapy, and on the central role of activity in the practice of occupational therapy.

Theories of human development recognise that life is characterised by a multitude of subtle transformations, some unique to the individual, and some general. Uniqueness (except in the case of monozygotic siblings) is, of course, established genetically at conception, and may be furthered by individualistic life experiences. Nevertheless, humans also have much in common, and some features of development appear to be universal. The human genetic make-up is quite different from that of other species, and all human cultures are based on regulations and expectations not found elsewhere in the animal kingdom. For this reason, many developmental theorists examine progress through the human lifespan in 'normative' terms. The advantage of this approach is that it offers a detailed description of age-related trends, thus providing a framework for considering the individual case.

Norms of human development are obtained through studying appropriate samples of people according to chosen criteria. Thus, Tanner (1963) chose to focus on physical correlates such as height and weight, while Gesell (1954) stressed maturational forces in drawing up behavioural norms for the early years of life. Other researchers have focused on cognitive trends, or on selected aspects of cognition, as did Kohlberg (1981) in his study of moral reasoning. To study a specific aspect of development in this way is largely a matter of convenience. Those who do so recognise that changes in one area have implications for others, and that human development is a holistic and integrated process. It is also a continuous one, in which changes do not appear abruptly; rather, each set of alterations builds upon previously established foundations, so that the process is often conceptualised as stage-like.

Occupational therapy gains its understanding of development from a number of disciplines, chiefly biology and psychology. The impact of biodevelopmental theories on the practice of occupational therapy has already been discussed and, in Chapter 3, readers were referred to primary sources of information in these areas. The present chapter will concentrate on cognitive and social development. In a book of this size, it is not possible to deal with all the issues that relate to these areas, so that only the most influential theories and studies will be covered. These will show that each developmental phase has it own norms, challenges and criteria of adjustment. It is important that therapists be aware of developmental milestones and typical modes of adjustment if they are to identify developmental deficits in the first place. Furthermore, intervention in the form of facilitating growth and development (for example, see Llorens 1968) is clearly impossible in the absence of a firm understanding of normal progress.

Maturation

Before actual theories of development are described, it should be noted that many of these incorporate the concept of *maturation*. This refers to the gradual unfolding of genetic influences, so that many facets of development, although not present at birth, remain under genetic control. Maturational theorists do not generally focus on individual differences in genetic make-up. Instead, they build their theories on the biological inheritance shared by all humankind and use this notion to account for regularities of development. Gesell (1954) is one such theorist, who has identified precise age-related correlates of growth in childhood. To the extent that maturation is uniform, his norms are reasonably accurate across cultures. Yet other theorists have offered slightly different age norms in respect of certain achievements. This does not mean that Gesell's norms deserve rejection. It simply indicates that while maturation remains perhaps the most important influence, other factors also enter the picture, principally individual predispositions and specific or cultural learning experiences. Norms, therefore, offer guidelines as to what we should expect in developmental terms, but they should not be interpreted too rigidly, certainly in respect of age limits.

Although biological maturation remains the chief influence on those aspects of development that are broadly age-related, there remains the fact that from the moment of conception individuals interact with their environment – be this the prenatal environment or the world of people and objects. The theories reviewed here are based on this concept of interaction. However, they are theories of normal development and are, therefore, more concerned with dimensions of the environment shared by the majority of people, than with circumstances that are unusual or traumatic.

COGNITIVE DEVELOPMENT: PIAGET'S THEORY

Jean Piaget (1896–1980) put forward a comprehensive theory of intellectual development which includes the concepts of *maturation*, *interaction* and *active learning*. According to Piaget, maturation limits the achievements of early childhood, and cognitive development proceeds in stages as biological capacity unfolds, that is, what the child can do is constrained by the degree of nervous system development. Thus, no matter the encouragement given, a 6-month-old child will not walk and likewise a 16-month-old child will not talk in sentences. The neonate has primitive cognitive structures, which are gradually elaborated as he begins to interact with the environment. Interaction is motivated by curiosity and the child's need to establish equilibrium between his understanding of the world and actual reality. Children are 'constructivist' in approach in the sense that they actively participate in their own mental development through manipulating objects, exploring the environment and attempting to solve problems. They are not simply passive recipients of facts.

Piaget's approach to intelligence differs from that of other theorists who share his interest in the topic. He is not concerned, as are the factor theorists, with subcomponents, nor is he concerned with individual differences. He equates intelligence with conceptual development, and his main concern is with the process of concept formation over time. In Piaget's view, concepts are the building blocks of knowledge. They aid our *adaptation* to the world since, to deal with the world about us, we need concepts, problem-solving abilities and rules of inference. We also need *operations*, which may be defined as internalised representations that are logical and reversible. Young children, however, do not have genuine operations, and Piaget discovered that their way of thinking is qualitatively different from that of adults. Children make many 'mistakes' of reasoning simply because their cognitive structures, or *schemata*, are not yet fully developed.

According to Piaget, a scheme is an organised representation of events. We do not merely react like automata to environmental stimuli; rather, we interpret what is happening according to schemata (or schemes). Schemata may be described as 'mental maps' of the world which grow and change over the years. Piaget postulates two biologically inherited processes to account for this change, namely *assimilation* and *accommodation*. He calls these 'functional invariants' because, although schemata may and do change, the processes which underlie cognitive development do not. Assimilation occurs when we incorporate new experiences into schemata that already exist, while accommodation involves changing or modifying ideas that are not fitted to some aspect of the environment. Clearly, the latter concept has much in common with Popper's notion that theories require modification if they fail to account for events.

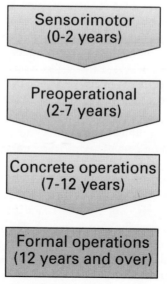

Fig. 4.1 Piaget's four stages of development.

Piaget divides the developmental process into four main stages (Fig. 4.1), some having further substages or phases. Children must pass through one stage before arriving at the next, and each new one builds upon foundations previously established. Piaget's stages span the period from birth to adolescence, and, throughout, intelligence develops through assimilation and accommodation. Our review will concentrate on the essential features of each stage, since detailed accounts are widely available elsewhere.

Box 4.1   Piaget's four stages of development

Sensorimotor stage (birth to 2 years)

The sensorimotor stage, which spans the period of infancy (from birth to 2 years of age), is characterised by exploratory actions. These are primitive at the outset and gradually develop until, towards the end of the stage, the infant's behaviour is purposeful and goal-directed. The sensorimotor period can be subdivided into a series of achievements. The neonate can only relate to objects through innate reflexes (e.g. sucking on a nipple), but, (1) within the first month, reflex-like actions appear in the absence of eliciting stimuli, and are practised spontaneously. (2) As more objects are incorporated into these reflexive schemata, the infant begins to organise sensory experiences and motor responses through a series of adaptive actions known as 'circular reactions'. Up to the age of 4 months, the infant repeats actions ('primary circular reactions') that centre on his own body and bring pleasurable results. (3) Thereafter (4–8 months), he repeats interesting actions that affect objects in the environment ('secondary circular reactions'). (4) Between 8 and 12 months, learned modes of action are combined and coordinated, and for the first time, the infant shows signs of intentional, means-end behaviour. At this stage, he also begins to imitate other people's actions. (5) Play becomes purposeful and experimental in the 'tertiary circular reactions' substage (12–18). At this time, the infant investigates all the possibilities for play inherent in some toy, and is no longer confined to reproducing formerly discovered effects. The actions are still circular because there is always some repetition of interesting results, but they are, at the same time, more varied and exploratory than ever before. (6) Finally, at the end of the sensorimotor period, attempts to solve simple problems are no longer tied to motor behaviour. Infants can now work out solutions mentally, as did Piaget's son, Laurent, when he saw a stick on a table and some tempting bread out of reach. He did not have to experiment with the stick in the trial-and-error fashion of the tertiary reactions substage, but could work out the answer before reaching for the stick and using it to draw the bread towards him. This sixth and final substage of the sensorimotor period, which lasts from roughly 18 months to 2 years of age, is entitled the 'invention of new means through mental combinations'.

In addition to the achievements outlined above, one other highly important concept evolves during the sensorimotor stage, that of object permanence. This refers to the child's understanding that objects have an independent existence and remain in the environment even when they cannot be seen. Infants under 4 months of age do not have this understanding. They may gaze at the spot where they last saw the object or person, but make no attempt to scan the environment. According to Piaget, they seem to relate the object's reappearance to their own gazing. Later, they may make crude, searching hand movements when an object falls from their grasp, but their focus is on their own actions, not on whatever has vanished from sight. Only at roughly 10 months of age, does purposeful searching begin for something that the infant has watched being hidden. However, he cannot yet track an object that may be hidden in two or more possible places, or one whose displacement he has not observed. The object concept is completed at 18 months. Now, instead of looking only at the place where the object was last seen, the infant can make inferences about where it might be.

For Piaget (1952), the achievements of the sensorimotor period provide evidence that human thought evolves from action. The infant begins life with reflexive, then behavioural schemata, and only at the end of the period does thought become symbolic. The infant's activities thus pave the way for the emergence of mental representations and simple problem-solving abilities.

Pre-operational stage (2 to 7 years)

The early part of the pre-operational stage (2–7 years) is marked by the enhancement of symbolic abilities, evident in the child's *pretend* play and use of words to represent events. Yet some aspects of thought remain primitive, for example animism, the belief that inanimate objects are alive. At the age of 4 years, the child enters the intuitive phase of the pre-operational stage, a phase which Piaget has described in great detail. He has shown principally that the child's thought at this stage is qualitatively different from that of older children and adults. In a series of experiments, Piaget found that pre-operational children find it difficult to classify objects or arrange a number of them in serial order (e.g. from largest to smallest). But his most famous experiments are those highlighting the child's inability to recognise that an object's properties remain unchanged when there is a superficial alteration in appearance. Piaget's experiments on the conservation of liquid are well-known, and take the following form: (1) The investigator displays two glasses of liquid; the glasses are the same size, and the child agrees there is an equal amount of liquid in each. (2) The contents of one are then poured into a taller vessel while the child watches. The pre-operational child will claim that there is 'more' liquid in the taller vessel. Piaget found that the child at this stage also has problems with the conservation of number, mass and area.

Piaget labels this stage 'pre-operational' because children in the age group do not have reversible representations and cannot retrace the steps that make up an action. Their judgements are based primarily on perceptual features, and they find it difficult to decentre – that is, to focus on more than one attribute at a time. In the liquid conservation problem, height alone is attended to, not height and width simultaneously. Piaget has also drawn attention to the child's egocentricity, or tendency to see the world from his own point of view, without regard to that of another.

Stage of concrete operations (7 to 12 years)

Concrete operational children have mastered the deficits of the previous stage. They understand the principles of class inclusion, relations (A is greater than B; B is greater than C: therefore A is greater than C) and conservation. Generally, conservation of number is acquired first – in fact towards the end of the pre-operational period – then that of mass and weight and, finally, volume (Tomlinson-Keasey et al 1979). The child can now represent a series of actions mentally, and can draw a map of some familiar route. However, thinking remains concrete in that reasoning is tied to familiar events and objects that are present. The child does not yet use algebra or abstract procedural rules. If asked to identify objects that will float in a basin of water, the concrete operational child tends to try one object after another, whereas older children will establish some sort of rule, such as 'all wooden objects float'. The child at this stage also finds it difficult to reason about abstract concepts (e.g. justice), and while he can reason about events that are happening or have happened, he cannot deal with hypothetical situations.

Stage of formal operations (12 years and beyond)

Formal operational thinking is systematic and abstract. The adolescent who has reached this stage of thought can reason about events that are logically possible, even if they are outside his experience of the real world. Thought is now adult-like, and in problem-solving the formal operator uses 'if/then' propositional statements, and tests out hypotheses systematically. Perhaps the best known experiment to illustrate the differences between concrete and formal reasoning is the 'four beaker and eyedropper' experiment, in which the child's task is to find out the liquids that, together with the chemical in the eyedropper, can be combined to produce a yellow colour. Children at the concrete stage typically mix the liquid in the eyedropper with that in each of the four glasses in turn, and then give up. Adolescents are much more systematic; they can generate a higher order procedural rule that takes every possible combination into account. On this basis, it does not take them too long to work out that if they mix the fluids in glasses one and three, and add the chemical in the eyedropper to this mixture, the desired yellow colour will result.

Criticisms of Piaget's theory

Piaget's influence on developmental psychology is second to none, yet he has his critics. Some have argued that his concept of age-related stages is too rigid; others that he underestimates the intelligence of younger children and overestimates that of adolescents.

Age-related stages

With respect to stages, it has been contended that changes in development do not occur quite so abruptly as Piaget claimed, and that the achievements that are supposed to characterise a given stage do not actually all appear simultaneously. Bower (1982), for example, argues that the object concept appears earlier than Piaget suggests, and he is critical of his 'searching' criterion; while others (for example Hunt 1976) claim that sensorimotor growth proceeds in at least 12 behavioural variants, as opposed to the six substages identified by Piaget. These researchers favour a continuous, gradual view of development, and it is for this reason that we have previously characterised development as 'stage-like'.

Intelligence of younger children

Critics who claim Piaget underestimates young children's intelligence often focus on the pre-operational stage. In this context, it has been argued that abilities tested according to a Piagetian format may misrepresent the child's real capacity, because the situation presented is unfamiliar and the language used too formal. Thus,

Gelman (1979) has found evidence of number conservation by 3-year-olds, and Donaldson (1978) has shown that, under appropriate conditions, pre-operational children are not necessarily egocentric. Others (for example Field 1981, May & Norton 1981) have indicated that training can accelerate pre-operational abilities; however, it must be admitted that findings in this area are not always consistent. Although many studies support the training perspective, there are at least as many that refute it, (for example Gruen 1965, Smedslund 1961) thereby supporting Piaget's biological thesis. One reason for this kind of inconsistency is that criteria for effective acceleration vary. Hughes & Noppe (1985) point out that all training studies should satisfy Piaget's three criteria for demonstrating that operational thought can be induced. These are:

1. that children must be able to explain how they solved the problem
2. the ability to solve the problems must persist over time
3. the children must be able to apply their newly learned solutions to other problems – that is, to generalise from one situation to another.

In these terms, it is evident that while many acceleration studies fulfil one, or maybe two of the necessary criteria, they fail to satisfy all three of the criteria in question. Thus far, no data have refuted Piaget's theory in toto, although they do suggest that it should be modified in a direction of continuous, stage-like development.

Intelligence of adolescents

The criticism that Piaget overestimates adolescent cognitive abilities arises from findings of considerable cognitive variation among this age group. It would appear that biological adolescence or, indeed, adulthood (Neimark 1979) does not guarantee formal operational thought, and Shaffer (1985) suggests that formal reasoning probably proceeds more gradually than is allowed for in the theory. In fact, Piaget never did claim that all formal abilities emerge simultaneously, and he has used the term 'décalage' to describe such non-uniformities of attainment. For any one cognitive stage, uneven patterns of development are said to reflect 'horizontal décalage' so that for the child reaching the formal period, 3 or 4 years will typically pass before logical, quasi-mathematical transformations are applied consistently to a variety of problems. Given this qualification, Piaget does hold the view that formal reasoning is fully developed by the middle years of adolescence. In effect, he sees no qualitative difference between the thinking processes of the adolescent and those of the mature adult, although there may be differences of content. For this reason, Piaget did not extend his theory to encompass the possibility of a level beyond formal operations. Recent work suggests this may be a shortcoming.

Cognition in adulthood

Evidence that cognitive development continues in adult life comes from many sources. One important source is the extensive set of results obtained by Lawrence Kohlberg on moral reasoning. Kohlberg has elaborated Piaget's early work on morality and, like Piaget, believes that changes in moral reasoning reflect more global advances in cognition. Using a system in which subjects are asked to resolve a series of moral dilemmas and give reasons for their answers, Kohlberg (1969) identified six stages of moral development. Later, he and his colleagues (Colby et al 1980) reported the results of a 20-year longitudinal study which found that adult subjects do reason at more advanced levels than their adolescent counterparts. These researchers found that the use of 'conventional reasoning' (stages 3 and 4) increased up to the age of 22, gradually displacing more primitive rationales. Subjects showed no evidence of 'postconventional reasoning' (stages 5 and 6) until they were in their early twenties and, even among 24-year-olds, only 10% of judgements were of this type. Kohlberg has concluded that, regardless of culture, only a small minority of adults is capable of reasoning at the highest level identified by him.

Just as researchers have found that conventional moral reasoning is the dominant mode within any society, research into other aspects of cognition supports the view that most adult thinking – at least in advanced societies – is characterised by the use of formal operations. However, some adults never use formal operations (Neimark 1979). While others – for example, Nobel prize-winners and the like – appear to operate on an even higher plane. If this is so, Piaget's assertion that formal operations constitute the 'final equilibrium', or the most mature possible form of reasoning, is seriously flawed. A number of investigators have, in fact, challenged this claim Patricia Arlin (1975, 1977) has voiced doubts about whether the thinking strategies of someone such as Einstein can validly be equated with those of a typical adolescent or young adult.

She contends that they cannot, and postulates a fifth stage of cognitive development, which she calls a *problem-finding* stage, describing Piaget's fourth stage as a *problem-solving* one. In her own work with university students, Arlin claims to have found results that validate her thesis. Almost half of her student sample approached problems in ways that demonstrated fifth-stage thinking, those advancing to this level being already formal operators.

It does seem to be the case that higher education fosters cognitive development beyond the formal-operational stage. Work by Commons and his associates (Commons et al 1982) indicates that postgraduates reason at more advanced levels than do undergraduates, and Commons insists that these differences are qualitative and not merely a reflection of horizontal décalage. In fact, he claims to have identified two stages beyond formal operations. The first is that of *systematic*, the second that of *metasystematic* reasoning. Commons and his colleagues found that a majority of postgraduates showed at least some evidence of systematic or metasystematic thinking, and that their performance was markedly superior to that of undergraduate students.

In summary, research into adult thinking suggests that some individuals do not reach the formal operational stage, and that some may advance beyond it. These variations were not predicted by Piaget and represent a flaw in his point of view. In common with a host of other developmental theorists, he has not given sufficient attention to the fact that development continues in adulthood; that it is, undeniably, a life-long process.

Implications of Piaget's theory for education

Although Piaget's theory is open to criticism in some respects, it remains influential and has had a great impact on early education. Educators now acknowledge that rote learning reveals little or nothing about a child's true understanding of a subject, and teaching today is geared to the pupil's developmental level and range of comprehension. Piaget's insistence that activity is central to the learning process is especially relevant to occupational therapy. While students at the formal-operational level may well be able to grasp abstract, verbally presented concepts, younger children, and those who are being taught some practical skill, learn best when the method of presentation is concrete and they are free to manipulate the tools of their task. Neo-Piagetian modifications further suggest that when we are teaching adults we should be aware that differing levels of reasoning may obtain among formal operators.

COGNITIVE DEVELOPMENT: LANGUAGE

All health professionals need some knowledge of their clients' level of linguistic ability. Although it is easy to identify obvious weaknesses – for instance in literacy and numeracy – others may be more elusive, yet equally important to identify and compensate for if a client is to follow and carry out instructions and express himself clearly.

Standardised tests

There are numerous tests of language on the market, many of which have a clinical focus; for example, tests geared to diagnosing articulation or comprehension difficulties, limitations of vocabulary and so forth. Many of these are standardised on random or stratified samples, or are at least semi-standardised in the sense that norms have been yielded by clinical populations. Although these tests are useful, they do pose problems because, having a narrow and specialised focus, they fail to capture the complexity and richness of natural language.

Experimental techniques

Another way of assessing language ability is to devise some kind of semi-experimental procedure. This is a popular method of assessing child language, and researchers often use it to develop age-related guides. With very young children, pictures, puppets and various toys have been used to assess comprehension of verb tenses, active versus passive statements and other aspects of syntax. For example, a child may be asked to demonstrate a toy mouse 'being chased' by a toy cat. An advantage of this technique is that it facilitates control of environmental variables from one child to another and the compilation of consistent results. A disadvantage is that the tests are administered in fairly artificial settings. Children may be inhibited under these conditions so that assessment may not reflect their true level of ability.

Analysis of spontaneous speech

Due to the limitations inherent in standardised tests and experimental techniques, several investigators have chosen to chart the course of normal language development by recording and analysing spontaneous speech. This approach is undoubtedly the best one to use with pre-school children. At this stage, the child's competence is more accurately expressed in speech when the child is playing in a familiar environment, with parents or siblings present, than when the child is merely responding to requests from an experimenter. It is not, however, an easy matter to chart language development in this way. The investigator must record a substantial corpus of child speech over frequent intervals and must take written notes of the context, where necessary, to facilitate interpretation. Thereafter, the researcher must transcribe and edit the great bulk of recorded material yielded, and devise a grammar to describe and summarise its basic structure and function. Given the heavy demands this method places on time and energy, investigators who use it typically focus on small samples of children. Within this tradition, the classical study is that of Roger Brown of Harvard University and his associates (Brown 1973; Box 4.2).

Box 4.2 Brown's (1973) study of early language development.

Brown investigated language development in three English-speaking children, Adam, Eve and Sarah, beginning his analysis at the point where they became capable of basic two-word combinations. He identified five early stages in all, each being characterised by an increase in MLU (mean length of utterance, measured in morphemes) and a particular line of advance not present in the preceding stage.

1. In the first stage, MLU is 1–2 morphemes, and the child uses what is aptly termed 'telegraphic' speech. For all its brevity, this kind of speech incorporates basic *semantic* and *grammatical* roles, such as *non-existence* (e.g. 'allgone milk'), *recurrence* ('more milk') and *possession* ('Adam ball').

2. The second stage (MLU 2–2.5 morphemes) is one in which meaning is modulated by the use of more appropriate word endings or inflections. Brown has identified 14 inflections which characterise stage 2 speech of children acquiring American English. Examples include the addition of *-ing* to verbs to form the present

progressive, the use of 's' to indicate plurals and possession, the inclusion of articles (both *a* and *the*) and mastery of the past tense.

3. Stage 3 (MLU 2.5–3.0) sees the formation of straightforward questions and negatives.

4. The child in the fourth stage (MLU 3.0–3.5) can use simple embedded sentences and subordinate clauses.

5. By stage 5 (MLU 3.5–4.0), speech has become quite sophisticated. There is now conjunction of simple sentences in which (a) subject or (b) predicate may be deleted as appropriate (e.g. (a) 'He's flying and swinging'; (b) 'You and I had some.').

Early language development

Several investigators have found that age is not the most reliable indicator of early language development, and it is for this reason that Brown preferred to use mean length of utterance (MLU). He observed that, in any event, complexity increases in line with MLU and that, even among his own three subjects, there were marked differences in the age at which they reached the various milestones, Eve being by far the most 'advanced' if one chooses to speak in these terms. Generally, children begin to combine words at around $1\frac{1}{2}$ to 2 years of age, but arrival at stage 5 may occur anywhere between 2 and $3\frac{1}{2}$ years. However, although language development is not closely tied to chronological age, its course of acquisition is remarkably regular. Infants from all cultures proceed from crying to cooing and then babbling, before they utter their first recognisable word, and patterns of consonant development are universal. The ability to comprehend others is generally more advanced than production abilities in the early stages, and early word combinations are invariably telegraphic. Slobin (1971) has studied stage 1 speech in several languages (including German, Russian, Finnish, Lao and Samoan) and concludes that all sampled utterances are similar to English in the basic semantic and grammatical relations they express. Although some children's speech may not reflect a particular relation or role (e.g. *action-locative* as in 'go car'), those that are expressed form a subset of the larger set identified by Brown.

Similarities of development across linguistic communities, together with children's astounding capacity to master a complex symbol system in a relatively short period of time, suggest the possibility of some innate biological predisposition that is specifically oriented to language. This possibility is strengthened by evidence for the notion that there is a 'critical period' for language development (Lenneberg 1967). Evidence is drawn, for the most part, from case studies which show that it is difficult for severely deprived children (e.g. 'feral' children) to acquire language if they are first exposed to it after puberty. However, the much publicised case of 'Genie' (Curtiss 1977), who at $13\frac{1}{2}$ years of age was released from the room in which she had been isolated since the age of 20 months, suggests that the term 'sensitive period' might be more appropriate. Genie did acquire a considerable working vocabulary, yet some 5 years after her rescue had an MLU of only 3, and her grasp of syntax remained greatly impoverished. She was, however, more advanced at the semantic level, and could carry out classification tasks appropriately (e.g. classification of objects and colours.)

Competence

It has been observed that what children actually acquire in the years up to puberty is *competence* in their native language. Chomsky (1965) has made a useful distinction between competence and *performance*. Performance relates to what is actually said in speech, while competence refers to the speaker's knowledge of the rules which govern sentence construction. Competence is therefore inferred from performance, since the person would be unable to devise sentences in the first place without a grasp of the underlying rules. This does not mean that a speaker's knowledge of the rules is conscious nor that he can articulate them fully. Certainly, a 5-year-old child is unlikely to offer a description of the structural procedures he is using to generate highly sophisticated sentences, and the same holds for most adults. It is, in fact, the job of the trained linguist to write a formal descriptive grammar of this kind. An interesting aspect of performance is that it is often severely flawed. Speakers may stutter, use tautologies and ungrammatical colloquialisms, pause in mid-sentence, or fail to complete what they intend to say. Yet young children acquire competence and fluency despite exposure to such an imperfect linguistic environment.

Clinical implications

The theoretical principles of developmental psycholinguistics (a fusion of linguistics and psychology) have important implications for clinical practice.

Implications for assessment

A knowledge of language development cautions us against making premature judgements about children's apparent linguistic impairment on the grounds of observed deficiencies in performance. Failure to recognise the distinction between competence and performance has resulted in sweeping general statements, such as those made by Basil Bernstein, a British sociologist writing in the 1960s and early 1970s. Bernstein (1967) claimed that typical social class differences in IQ were due largely to differences in the language codes used, lower socio-economic groups using a *restricted* code, and middle class groups an *elaborated* one. Restricted codes use short, simple sentences, are limited in precision, and are closely tied to context. Elaborated language is more complex and differentiated and can express a wider range of thoughts. Bernstein proposed that elaborated codes orient children to abstract thinking, whereas children whose parents use a restricted code are oriented towards concrete, less conceptual thinking. As an example, a father using a restricted code might tell his child to eat up. The child says, 'Why?' and the father replies, 'Because I told you so', or 'Because I'm in a hurry'. An elaborated reply might involve telling the child that food is necessary for growth, or even, 'Because food has vitamins, darling, and you need vitamins to grow'.

Although Bernstein's thesis has initial, commonsense appeal, it overlooks the fact that people may use a particular code on grounds of custom or social acceptability, yet have access to a more complex code when the situation is appropriate. Most of us, in any event, do switch codes in this way, for example, when writing to a friend as against writing an academic essay. Labov's study (1970) of black, New York ghetto children emphasises this point. In one case study, a young subject who used a highly restricted code when first interviewed became relaxed and much more fluent on a second, informal occasion. This was deliberately set up to resemble a 'chat' more than an interview, and the subject's best friend was also present.

Implications for teaching methods

While studies of language development further imply that children do not need formal teaching to acquire syntax, educators of very young children should keep some basic principles in mind. Firstly, the speech that young subjects hear about them should be closely tied to meaning. Parents seem to recognise this intuitively when they use gesture and intonation to emphasise the relationship between sound and significance. Secondly, language acquisition is not a passive process. Children are prompted to speak by their need to communicate, and Snow and coworkers (Snow et al 1976) have found that children do not acquire language (in this case, a foreign one) simply by watching television. The give and take of conversation, however primitive, appears to be a prerequisite. Thirdly, although minimal teaching appears to be all that is necessary for competence, evidence from sociolinguistics indicates that if the right conditions are met (as in Labov's study), educators can achieve a closer match between competence and performance in subjects who are deprived or who suffer developmental deficits.

Occupational therapists are ideally placed to incorporate these principles into their teaching methods. They may devise activities that are centred on a requirement to communicate, or develop games to facilitate fluency; for example, 'reading the news on television' to an audience of peers. Finally, children can be taught a great deal about *pragmatics*. This aspect of language refers to *how* language should be used in different situations. It involves norms of politeness, and taking into account the status of the person being addressed. Piaget (1959) has also pointed out that children's speech is often inappropriate in that much of it is *egocentric*. Egocentric speech assumes no difference between the speaker's perspective and that of the listener. Educators can devise situations to modify these tendencies, just as they can teach subjects how to make polite and appropriate requests. In the case of older children, social skill training procedures that are traditionally used with adults, can be adapted and modified as required.

PSYCHOSOCIAL DEVELOPMENT (Boxes 4.3–4.5)

CRISIS PERIODS OF ADULTHOOD

Several investigators have been inspired by Erikson's work to study the stages of adulthood more extensively, while adhering to his thesis that each phase focuses on some particular developmental crisis; for example, Gould (1978) considers that the middle years can be just as stressful as those of adolescence. The better-known studies

Contd on page 98

Box 4.3 Psychosocial development: Freud's stages

According to Sigmund Freud, psychosocial and psychosexual development are closely intertwined. Human development, in his view, is largely a matter of learning how to manage and direct the instinctual energy of the libido in appropriate ways; likewise the aggressive instinct. Since instincts create tension, and since tension reduction occurs in a context of people and cultural constraints, psychosexual, psychosocial and personality development are inevitably one and the same. Freud further believed that psychosexual development proceeds in stages, whose roots can be traced to early infancy (Table 4.1) – a belief that was highly controversial in his day.

Table 4.1 Freud's stages of psychosexual development

Age (years)	Stage
0–1	Oral
1–3	Anal
3–6	Phallic
6–12	Latency
12 onwards	Genital

Oral stage

The first stage described by Freud is the oral stage (birth to 1 year), during which libidinal energy is focused on the mouth, and gratification is sought through sucking, chewing and similar oral activities.

Anal stage

In the anal stage (1–3 years), libido concentrates in the anal region. Just as weaning can create tensions in the previous stage, toilet training may now be a source of frustration and conflict.

Phallic stage

The phallic stage (3–6 years) is one in which the child

becomes capable of sexual arousal. According to psychoanalytic theory, the child at this stage is attracted to the parent of the opposite sex, and at the same time feels threatened by the same-sex parent, who is seen as a hostile rival. In the case of the boy, this 'Oedipus complex' is successfully resolved if, instead of trying to possess his mother exclusively, he tries to win her affections indirectly. He does this by identifying with his father, a solution which also helps to reduce his 'castration anxiety'. The analagous, though less dramatic, conflict for the girl is termed the 'Electra complex'. Undoubtedly the most important outcome of this period is the establishment of gender identity. The boy who identifies with his father imitates his behaviour and internalises his attitudes and values, making them his own. In much the same manner, the mother becomes a role model for her daughter, who internalises 'feminine' values and sex-role expectations. During the phallic period, the superego emerges and puts added pressure on the child to become more fully socialised.

Latency stage

The latency stage (6–12 years) brings with it a diffusion of libido and a decline in sexual interest which last until puberty.

Genital stage

At puberty, the individual reaches the final genital stage of development, wherein sexual strivings are acknowledged and, ideally, are managed in a socially responsible way.

Freud's theory is centred on the principle that childhood profoundly influences the adult personality. This influence may be benign, giving rise to a rational, ego-controlled mode of adjustment in later life, but all too often it is not. Where there are severe and only partially resolved conflicts at any one stage, development may be arrested or 'fixated' at that point. Thus, unresolved oral conflicts are reflected in the adult 'oral character' who is prone to overeating or heavy smoking. Fixation at the phallic stage may result in homosexuality, or in doubts about sexual identity, leading to promiscuity in order to affirm it. Because Freud believed that biological forces and childhood experiences are the prime (albeit unconscious) motivators of adult behaviour, he has often been labelled a determinist.

Box 4.4 Psychosocial development: Erikson's theory

Erik Erikson's account of psychosocial development is more comprehensive than Freud's, in that he recognises and delineates several adult phases of growth. Although Erikson's theory is grounded in psychoanalytic thinking, he places greater stress than did Freud on the influence of specific cultures and on the role of the ego. Erikson believes that human beings are rational creatures who need to develop effective means of adapting to sociocultural demands. These demands vary throughout life, and, accordingly, Erikson has identified eight phases of development (Table 4.2). To the extent that each stage incorporates some characteristic conflict between self and society, each represents a crisis period in the individual's

Table 4.2 Erikson's eight stages of psychosocial development*

Developmental stage	Psychosocial crisis	Positive outcome
1. **Early infancy**	Basic trust v. Mistrust	Drive and hope
2. **Late infancy**	Autonomy v. Shame or doubt	Self-control
3. **Early childhood**	Initiative v. Guilt	Purpose
4. **Middle childhood/Latency**	Industry v. Inferiority	Method and competence
5. **Puberty and adolescence**	Identity v. Role confusion	Devotion and fidelity
6. **Young adulthood**	Intimacy v. Isolation	Affiliation/love
7. **Mid-adulthood**	Generativity v. Stagnation	Care
8. **Maturity and old age**	Ego integrity v. Despair	Renunciation and wisdom

* Adapted from Erikson (1963)

life. Failure to resolve a developmental crisis typically creates adjustment problems at some future stage, but Erikson is optimistic about human resourcefulness. In particular, he holds that those who solve a specific life-crisis successfully are better equipped to manage conflicts that may occur at some future stage. In this sense, life crises are not construed as negative events. Rather, they are viewed as positive forces for growth.

Conflicts of adolescence

According to Erikson's account of development, the person who has successfully surmounted the crises of childhood is one who has learned to trust others and feels capable of autonomous action and initiative. Social relationships and academic challenges during the *industry versus inferiority* period will – where the outcome is favourable – have affirmed a sense of self-worth, and the individual is now ready to grapple with the conflicts of adolescence. The adolescent's most important quest is for a sense of personal identity, and one way to achieve this is to experiment with the great number of social and occupational roles available. Experimentation offers opportunities for testing out values, capabilities, likes and dislikes – all of which pertain to self-concept development. However, the period is a lengthy one, and there are many choices to be made. Some adolescents do not succeed in finding social and vocational roles that are compatible with what they want out of life and, in consequence, they may enter adulthood experiencing 'identity confusion'. Erikson has pointed out that a great deal of adolescent rebelliousness can be traced to the conflicts of this period and the need to avoid confusion.

James Marcia (1966) has affirmed the value of crisis in adolescence (Box 4.5). Defining crisis as a period of choosing between meaningful alternatives, he concludes that to arrive at a mature status of 'identity achieved', the adolescent must have experienced both a crisis *and* a commitment to some course of action. Those who have experienced neither, can achieve only an 'identity diffused' status, whereas commitment without crisis results in 'identity foreclosure' – a situation that often coincides with personal immaturity. Adolescents in the throes of a crisis, who have yet to make a commitment, have a 'moratorium status', Experience of moratorium is a necessary prelude to acquiring maturity of identity.

Box 4.5   Marcia's four statuses of identity

Adolescents and young adults in the *identity diffused* category are those who are experiencing what Erikson (1968) terms 'role confusion'. Generally they lack vocational direction and a secure sense of self, have poorly developed political and ideological values and may appear to be floundering. According to Marcia (1966, 1980) identity diffusion is likely where the person has not explored meaningful alternatives (that is, has not experienced a crisis) and has not made a commitment to a set of actions or goals. For Marcia, commitment implies a degree of personal investment in what one is doing or plans to do.

Identity foreclosure occurs when the person has made a commitment but has not experienced a crisis. Adolescents in this category tend to accept parental values uncritically. They frequently allow adults to make educational and vocational decisions on their behalf, and may have had few opportunities to explore the various roles and options available.

Adolescents experiencing a *moratorium status* are in the throes of a crisis, but have yet to commit themselves. They are actively querying prevailing values and exploring worthwhile alternatives with a view to eventual commitment. Some researchers have found that college attendance increases the likelihood of moratorium status (e.g. Waterman & Waterman 1972), since undergraduates are encouraged to assess received opinion critically and rethink their vocational aspirations.

An *identity achieved* status reflects the experience of crisis and the fact that the individual has made enduring commitments. Nevertheless, Marcia (1980, pp 60–61) cautions that resolution of the identity conflict in adolescence does not guarantee an end to all problems. Identity development is a life-long processs, and a well-developed identity is flexible: 'It is open to changes in society and to changes in relationships. This openness assures numerous reorganizations of identity *contents* throughout th "identity-achieved" person's life, although the essential identity *process* remains the same, growing stronger through each crisis.'

of early and middle adulthood tend to be descriptive, rather than explanatory (as indeed is Erikson's own account); as with Gould's review, they eschew statistical analysis and are often based on interviews and biographical data. For this reason, results may not be generalisable. Nevertheless a number of qualitative analyses are admirably thorough, and have yielded valuable insights into this part of the lifespan.

A particularly influential account of adult development is that of Daniel Levinson (1978) in his book *The Seasons of a Man's Life*. As the title suggests, his focus is on male development. His sample was made up of 40 American male interviewees, born in the 1920s, who provided biographical histories. Levinson analysed this material, concentrating on data indicative of common patterns of change. On this basis, he concluded that each five-year period, from late adolescence to age 65, constitutes a developmental period in its own right. However, that of 'entering the adult world' (age 22–28 years) lasts for six years, and another phase, termed 'settling down', lasts for seven years, from age 33 to 40 years.

Levinson is most interested in mid-life adjustment. His subjects happened to be middle-aged at time of interview, so that his data for this stage are more reliable than are those pertaining to earlier phases, which are based on retrospective accounts. According to his description, men typically reach the point of entry to middle age at roughly 40 years of age. This milestone is preceded by early adulthood, whose chief characteristic is an 'age 30 transition', followed by the 'settling down' period. During the age 30 transition, subjects are chiefly concerned with establishing themselves in the world of work. This can be a demanding period, requiring years of training or further study. The person may stick to the career path he chose in his twenties, or may experiment with alternatives, even to the extent of changing his line of work. Whatever he does, he is mainly striving to establish a secure occupational identity. The mid-life transition period (40–45 years) is generally one of considerable conflict, suggesting that the term 'mid-life crisis' is an apt one. Levinson found that 80% of his sample experienced 'tumultuous struggles within the self and with the external world' at this time. Many reported dissatisfaction with wives and families, and some felt equally constrained by superiors and colleagues at work. Typically, this stage involves a change in time perspective. There is less reflection on the past, and greater recognition that time left in the future is limited and that goals may remain unfulfilled.

As people settle into middle age, they become more realistic in their expectations. Most men have reached the highest peak of their careers at this stage, and investigations which include female subjects (e.g. Havighurst 1982) show that this is also likely to hold true for women with unbroken career records. Many married women, having given up their jobs to rear children, successfully return to work in their forties. For Erikson, the period of middle adulthood, from 40 to 65 years, is one in which the healthy individual shows care and concern for the next generation. He points out (Erikson 1963) that older people need the young, every bit as much as children depend upon adults. Adults who do not concern themselves with influencing a younger generation may feel a sense of futility and selfish stagnation.

Critique of the stage view of adult development

Not all experts agree with the authorities quoted above on the near-inevitability of crisis at various points of development. Neugarten (1970) claims that crises do not relate to developmental stages, but to the occurrence of life-events that are not anticipated, or that are perceived as inappropriate to a particular epoch of the lifespan. Others challenge the conventional wisdom that adolescence or the mid-life transition are especially likely to be characterised by stress (e.g. Offer & Offer 1975). It has further been argued that the stage approach places too great an emphasis on personality change, and ties these changes too closely to chronological age. Against this, there is evidence that personality remains remarkably stable over the adult years (Costa & McCrae 1980). The consistency-change debate, however, largely reflects differences in methodology employed. Personality researchers tend to use standardised measures of traits, such as Cattell's 16 PF inventory (Siegler et al 79), while stage theorists use unstructured questionnaires or biographical information (Gould 1978, Levinson 1978). In any case, those who report an overall picture of stability admit to high levels of change in some personality attributes (e.g. Schaie & Parham 1976), although they are more likely to locate the cause in sociocultural events. A criticism of both the stage and life-events perspectives is that neither takes the issue of individual differences sufficiently into account. Events that are stressful for some may not be so for others. And where events are clearly traumatic enough to merit the label 'crisis', some people are better able than others to manage the situation.

The overall picture of development from childhood to middle adulthood appears to be one of overall stability, characterised, at the same time, by elements of change. This picture is consistent with both the stage and life-events approaches and, indeed, corresponds to our own experience of adulthood. We do not expect family members or friends to change radically to the extent that their behaviour is erratic and unpredictable from one year to the next, or even from one decade to another. Yet we expect some change, for we assume that people learn and profit from the experiences of life; indeed, not to do so implies an unhealthy rigidity. Lifespan changes reflect many influences. They reflect biological ageing, adjustments to social circumstances, the impact of specific experiences and individualistic interpretations of these events and reactions to them. Stability reflects our common biological inheritance and the fact that a great deal of social experience is regular from culture to culture. Moreover, development is guided by well-recognised, probably universal, human needs. These range from the biological needs identified by Freud and various drive theorists, to the higher level needs identified by Maslow and his humanistic colleagues. Certainly, the need to stabilise the self-concept and achieve self-actualisation is a recurrent theme in studies of adolescent and adult development. Human beings acquire strategies for fulfilling their needs, and to the extent that these are successful, they will be employed fairly consistently throughout life. Methods of meeting basic needs and identity needs – be they personal or vocational – will not be easily abandoned if they have proved effective in the past. Yet, the psychologically healthy individual is flexible enough to vary strategies of problem-solving where specific situations call for change. There is, then, agreement between stage and non-stage theories that overcoming problems at one point in life facilitates problem-solving and adjustment in the future.

Implications for practice

A knowledge of normal development brings several benefits to practice. First and foremost, it reminds us that every transition phase is characterised by its own set of needs and modes of adaptation, and that trauma or incapacity does not change this aspect of development. People remain human, with normal human requirements, even in the face of considerable adversity. There is, too, the fact that many basic skills are acquired in the years prior to adulthood. This is particularly the case for the skills needed for functional living. However, many clients who present at therapy experience developmental deficits. A knowledge of the normal developmental process enables the occupational therapist to identify these, and plan a programme of intervention around the developmental tasks that need to be mastered.

LATE ADULTHOOD

For Erikson, the eighth and final stage of development lasts from 65 years of age onwards, and its characteristic conflict is that of ego integrity versus despair. It is, according to him, a time wherein retrospection comes again to the fore. Adjustment is governed by whether the person considers that his or her life has been well-spent or disappointing, for in this phase the individual's outlook will generally be either positive or negative. It should be remembered that the final phase of life remains a developmental one. It is not merely a static period of looking back over the past, but also one in which the person may look forward to enjoying the fruits of retirement.

There is a sense in which the stage of late adulthood has been presented more negatively than is actually warranted. Clinical textbooks frequently focus on undesirable and often atypical correlates of ageing. Thus, we read of inevitable physical and psychological incapacity, hearing and sight loss, incipient or actual dementia and the like. While growing old does increase the likelihood of chronic and debilitating disorders, these are not inevitable concomitants and may well reflect negligence or misuse. Obviously a long history of, say, smoking, drinking to excess, or following a poor diet, is more likely to contribute to disease than is a short one. Diseases that are more common in the elderly include arthritis, diabetes, heart disease, emphysema and hypertension – all of which are known to relate in some way to environmental factors. One problem about conducting research on the elderly is that participating subjects may be suffering from one or more of the more common ailments. The variables of age and ill-health are therefore confounded. Results which purport to reflect some aspect of the *normal* ageing process, actually reflect the contribution of disease as well.

As is well known, the number of people who survive to a 'ripe old age' is increasing, at least in more prosperous countries where there have been marked advances in health-care and nutrition. The 1980 US census showed that 11.3% of the American population was over age 65; this figure is expected to reach 18% by the year 2030. Meanwhile in Britain, there are well over 2000 centenarians – a ten-fold increase over the past 30 years (Walmsley & Margolis 1987). Since women have a longer life expectancy than men, the ratio of women to men increases with age. Davison & Neale (1986) report a ratio in the United States of 125 women to 100 men between the ages of 65 to 69 years; for people aged 85 and over, the ratio is 229 females to 100 males.

Physical changes

Biological ageing principally brings changes in the musculoskeletal, cardiovascular, respiratory and sensory systems of the body. Related to these is a decline in muscular strength and perceptual acuity, and greater rigidity of posture. As muscles atrophy, surrounding tissues become flabby. Bones lose their density and the risk of osteoporosis and fracture is increased. The skin loses its elasticity. Deteriorations in the immune system make the older individual more likely to develop disease in response to stress. Within the brain, neurons decrease in number and there may be a degree of atrophy. At sensory levels, hearing and visual defects are most pertinent to daily living tasks. A characteristic hearing impairment is the inability to perceive high-frequency sounds. Visually, the lens of the eye yellows, becomes opaque and less accomodating: acuity diminishes and there is greater sensitivity to glare. The onset of these changes, however, is gradual. They normally begin in middle age but do not actually start to affect daily functioning until the person has reached his seventies or eighties. For these and other reasons, investigators of late adulthood generally make a distinction between the young-old and the old-old. The first group contains people aged between 65 and 74 years; the old-old category contains people aged 75 years and older. Flanagan (1981) interviewed 1000 people in the young-old age-group, their ages ranging from 68 to 72 years. Only 30% of the sample reported fair or poor health, and only 6% reported their health to be in the poor category.

Psychological changes

Investigations of psychological changes in the elderly generally report deficits in IQ, in problem-solving abilities and in memory. With respect to intelligence, performance IQ tends to decline, while indices of verbal intelligence show less deterioration, excepting abilities for mental arithmetic and abstract reasoning. In problem-solving, flexibility and creativity tend to decrease, and more time is needed to perform various psychomotor tasks. Studies of memory indicate that short-term retention is more apt to be affected by ageing than memory for less recent events. Short-term retention is most affected when the material to be learned needs to be reorganised. For example, when subjects are asked to repeat a list of digits in reverse order, performance declines with age, but the effects are far less for immediate recall without reversal (Bromley 1988). Vocabulary appears to be fairly resistant to ageing, certainly in those of above average intelligence. Research into other aspects of memory has produced contradictory results. These are due in part to variations in assessment measures used, but other variables may also account for inconsistent findings. Firstly, elderly participants in research may be on some kind of medication that induces retrieval failure. Secondly, they may be unused to having to encode or 'chunk' material, and often there is an improvement in test-performance when they are instructed how to do so (Hultsch 1971). Thirdly, individual differences in ability can influence results. Cavanaugh (1983) found that subjects over 65 years who had good vocabularies, could remember more about recently viewed television programmes than could their peers or younger subjects with poor verbal ability.

Social aspects of ageing

Throughout the western world, 65 years is arbitrarily set as the age at which most non-self-employed people retire. It is, of course, an average age. Numerous people retire earlier and many continue to work for far longer, often on a part-time basis (see Ch. 9).

Disengagement theory v. activity theory

Retirement brings with it a major social change. The person is no longer bound by a routine and there is loss of contact with work colleagues. Often, retired individuals enjoy their increased leisure at the outset, but after a 'honeymoon' phase, disenchantment sets in. There may be a tendency gradually to see friends less and less frequently, and to withdraw from personal contacts. *Disengagement theory* is an attempt to account for the older person's decreased interest in social affairs. The theory was developed by Cumming & Henry (1961), who argued that disengagement is a mutual process of withdrawal: not only does the individual lose interest in society, but society ceases in turn to concern itself with the ageing person. Curiously, Cumming & Henry claim this is an admirable development. They hold that disengagement and self-preoccupation increase satisfaction and are beneficial for adjustment. In any event, they see the process as inevitable.

The implications of disengagement theory have been widely researched but not very widely upheld. For example, the theory predicts that those who disengage most will be happiest, but this has not received substantial support (Maddox 1968, Reichard et al 1962). Nor is it true that disengagement is inevitable. Maddox (1964) found wide variations in patterns of withdrawal among older subjects, many of whom led very active lives. In opposition to disengagement theory, *activity theory* posits that high levels of involvement and activity benefit adjustment and satisfaction in later life. Again, tests of this theory have achieved mixed results (Mindel & Vaughan 1978, Neugarten et al 1968). In Neugarten's (1968) study, she and her colleagues identified four personality types within late adulthood, and found that the main differences in life satisfaction were between those who were active and involved, who appeared the most satisfied group, and those she called 'passive-dependent and unintegrated types', who were least active and involved, and least satisfied with life.

It would appear then that among people aged 65 years and older, some prefer the satisfactions offered by disengagement, while others prefer to involve themselves in activity. Atchley (1976) found that among retired males, teachers were more likely to 're-engage' themselves in social activities than were males of lower socio-economic status. Activity theory stresses this 'role-count' aspect of adjustment. It suggests that where the roles of middle-life cannot be maintained, substitute roles, appropriate to the person's age should be sought.

Chronological v. psychological age

Chronological age is not the best indicator of psychological ageing. Many individuals in science, politics and the arts have made major contributions in their various fields over the age of 65. Yet society, and the elderly themselves, often have negative perceptions of this stage in life. Santrock & Bartlett (1986) make the point that western cultures have a more negative stereotype of the aged than do Asian and other cultures; this may affect expectations about roles. Dyson (1980) contends that the disengagement/activity debate may have a political dimension. Emphasis on social withdrawal may reflect society's values regarding the elderly; it suits the social system to assume that disengagement is a 'sociological given' and that is also both beneficial and satisfying. Dyson proposes that it might be more enlightening to think of the situation within a social exchange framework. In this, the relationship between the individual and society is one in which the older person receives a pension and increased leisure time in return for leaving the work force and vacating extra places. On the surface this exchange appears to be equitable, but it may be achieved at considerable psychological cost. Furthermore, the individual who is himself a member of society and as such accepts its values, may feel guilt or discomfort if inclined to question the fairness of the exchange. Dyson argues that non-superficial investigations of retirement must take these issues into account.

Research into late adulthood

Although various programmes have been set up in the United States to examine the effects of exercise, nutrition and stimulation on ageing (Walmsley & Margolis 1987), there is a dearth elsewhere of research on late adulthood, relative to that on other stages in life. In his article, 'The neglect, of the elderly by British Psychologists', Bender (1986) highlights the importance of drawing attention to this age-group – in particular to its disabled and disadvantaged members – since public awareness influences the allocation of funds. Nevertheless, he points out, the elderly receive little or no attention in influential journals. 'Thus', he writes, 'the 15% of the population over 65 are almost totally ignored'. Bender's comments are based on a 2-year review of mainstream British psychological journals, all of which have clinical, social or medical issues as a main focus. He reviewed 264 papers in all and found that only nine of these focused on the elderly. Where articles concentrated on some general topic, only 26 subjects over 65 were included. And where an article did pertain to late adulthood, emphasis was invariably on pathology, focusing on such aspects as incontinence, amnesia and dementia. Clearly, according to Bender, the elderly do not think. The sole study of non-pathological cognitive functioning was carried out in Melbourne, Australia by Smith & Brewer (1985), and concerned itself with reaction time. Likewise, studies of normal functioning in social and other areas were more likely to come from non-British authors.

Undoubtedly, we need to know more about the normal ageing process. While it is well known that health and income are the two most important determinants of satisfaction in old age, there remains a gap between public perceptions of adjustment criteria at this stage and the experience of people within the age-group. American research indicates that public expectations are more negative than is warranted. For example, 65% of people under 65 years expect older persons to be lonely, whereas only 13% of older adults report loneliness to be a problem. Similar trends pertain in regard to expectations about health, income and fear of crime (e.g. Harris 1975). In fact, Harris' study found that the main worry reported by older people centred on the high cost of energy. This is not a problem highlighted in the literature, yet 42% of subjects reported it as one. In contrast, only 21% of older subjects reported health as a significant problem.

One variable insufficiently researched, insofar as it may influence late adulthood adjustment, is that of education. Its role in studies to date has been relatively understated, simply because previous generations have not been educated to the extent that has prevailed in recent decades. Cohort studies, which compare subjects across generations, have not taken this difference into account. It may well be that older adults of current and future generations have, for the first time in their lives, the chance to put their education to use in personal (as opposed to job-related) pursuits. This aspect of ageing will pertain more to women than to men, since women live longer and are also better educated than have been previous generations of women.

It may also be the case that studies in the future which control for educational levels will find few distinguishing differences between males and females in old age. It has already been found that characteristics which supposedly differentiate between the sexes do not, in fact, do so, at least in middle age. For example, the *empty nest* syndrome is supposed to be more characteristic of women than men – women are expected to feel devastated when their children leave home and they no longer have a clear purpose to their lives. However, the reality is quite different. In fact, both parents experience feelings of pronounced relief (Harkins 1978, Pearlin & Radabaugh 1979) when their mature offspring eventually decide to depart. There are currently several popular myths pertaining to sex differences among elderly couples. One is that women are likely to be irritated by retired, role-deprived men who lounge about and interfere with female housekeeping 'duties'. Given that males of recent decades are more likely to have shared in household tasks, particularly in dual-career families, future research will probably fail to identify sex-role differences of this kind.

THE INFLUENCE OF DEVELOPMENTAL THEORIES ON OCCUPATIONAL THERAPY PRACTICE

In Chapter 3, it was suggested that the theoretical base for the practice of occupational therapy is derived from three sources: the basic sciences, theories of human development and an understanding of the role of activity both in promoting health and in treating illness. It is reasonable to suggest, therefore, that theories of human development have had a profound influence on existing frames of reference for the practice of occupational therapy. These developmental theories attempt to describe and explain events which themselves are not visible as they occur at a sub-cortical, automatic or unconscious level. However, evidence of successful and integrated development is made visible through motor activity and other forms of behaviour. An individual's activity is both a tool for development and the evidence of development (Fig. 4.2). It is an understanding of this dual role of activity that offers occupational therapy its uniqueness of practice. Each of the frames of reference identified in Chapter 3 relates to some aspect of development. Each recognises that interruptions to the normal developmental processes may be caused by trauma of a physical or psychosocial nature, and each suggests that remedial intervention may occur through the use of activity as a learning experience for the promotion of change.

Adaptive performance

The frame of reference based on adaptive performance seeks to intervene and help the client overcome developmental deficits in the sub-skills needed for competent 'doing'.

Frame of Reference	Deficit
1 Adaptive performance	Competent 'doing'
2 Understanding of development	In some aspect of human development
3 Understanding of sensory integration	Trauma to the sensory-integrative process
4 Cognitive development	Satisfactory lifestyle with permanent impairment
5 Understanding of general systems theory	Developmental insufficiencies in role performance
6 Rehabilitation	Developmental interruptions, physical and psychosocial, due to trauma or illness

Fig. 4.2   The influence of developmental theories on practice.

Fidler, writing on adaptive performance as a frame of reference for the practice of occupational therapy, leans heavily on the developmental stages identified by Freud and the crisis resolution sequences suggested by Erikson. Fidler suggests that fixation at a particular developmental stage and/or non-resolution of a developmental crisis will be made evident through the problem-solving style of an individual, as evidenced in an attempt to perform a simple, concrete task. The value of the concrete task is that it remains present and apparent for the individual attempting it. Individuals may then recognise their own pattern of problem-solving, and possibly seek to change this to a more successful one. For example: they may be unwilling to attempt the task at all without minute, step-by-step instruction and support from the occupational therapist (who thus becomes the 'problem solver'); they may be unwilling to proceed and complete the task, constantly seeking 'perfection'; they may address a simple task in a way which makes it so complex that the task is virtually impossible to achieve; or they may repeatedly postpone progress while seeking unneeded and unavailable tools or materials. Within a group, collectively engaged in a simple task, individuals are required to contribute their own problem-solving skills in a cooperative or collaborative way. This is a higher order requirement than obtains when working alone, but it also provides opportunities for an inspection of interactive behaviour, in which the client may appear inhibited or destructive, be seen to ignore the needs and contributions of others in the group. Mosey extended Fidler's ideas when she suggested that these same techniques could be used to provide the opportunity for the 'recapitulation of ontogenesis', the chance to go back and try again, to develop more successful problem-solving skills and thus to resolve the developmental crisis in a more positive way. This frame of reference focuses on the individual's recognition of his own developmental deficit, the identification of the developmental stage of fixation or unresolved crisis, and then on the client's attempt to move on more successfully through the developmental process.

Developmental

The frame of reference based on an understanding of development in both a horizontal and a longitudinal aspect seeks to intervene and help the client to overcome deficits in his or her development. In the initial presentation of this frame of reference, Llorens (1970) suggests that:

Occupational therapy, through the skilled application of activities and relationships, can provide growth and development links to assist in closing the gap between expectations and ability.

and that:

Occupational therapy, through the skilled application of activities and relationships, can provide growth experiences to prevent the development of potential maladaptation.

Llorens thus suggests the application of this frame of reference for both intervention and prevention.

The rationale for a developmental frame of reference for the practice of occupational therapy is identified by Tiffany (1977) as follows:

1. human beings develop in a sequential way
2. each new gain in structure (physical or mental) enables the individual to gain in function
3. each new gain in functional ability makes further development and adaptation possible
4. physical, sensory, perceptual, cognitive, social and emotional aspects of the individual are intimately connected and affect the developmental state of the *whole* individual

5. conditions of stress cause the individual to regress to earlier levels of adaptation
6. successful experiences foster a sense of wholeness and competence.

Sensorimotor

The frame of reference based on an understanding of sensory integration seeks to intervene and help the client to overcome developmental insufficiences due to trauma to the sensory integrative process. Ayres and others have written extensively on this frame of reference and the theories upon which it relies, and they are not discussed again here. It is simply noted that a thorough understanding of the process by which vestibular, proprio-adaptive and tactile sensations are integrated within the nervous system so that adaptive motor responses may occur is vital for the implementation of this frame of reference.

Cognitive

The frame of reference based on cognitive development uses a somewhat different approach. Allen suggests that, as cognitive abilities are often permanently impaired in many chronic conditions, the role of the occupational therapist is to measure the residual cognitive level and so to intervene by assisting the individual in the pursuit of a satisfactory life style within these limitations. However, a secure grasp of normal cognitive development is a prerequisite for the implementation of this frame of reference.

Role performance

The frame of reference based on an understanding of general systems theory seeks to intervene and help the client to overcome developmental insufficiencies in role performance. This particular frame of reference was initially postulated by Reilly, who suggested that the roles of human beings could be seen as an attempt to master the environment in which they live. Barris and Kielhofner have written extensively on ways in which the concept of role performance may be used as a framework for inspecting the functional competence of clients. Appropriate roles and the developmental maturation needed both to identify necessary roles and to perform then adequately is a function of normal development, which may be hindered by environmental factors. The attempt to identify, inspect and overcome these factors forms the major thrust of occupational therapy intervention premissed on this particular frame of reference.

Rehabilitation

The frame of reference based on rehabilitation seeks to intervene and help the client to overcome developmental interruptions due to trauma and/or illness in both the physical and psychosocial domains. Both illness and trauma may deprive the individual of once-attained developmental status. The ability to perform the tasks needed for self-maintenance, work or leisure may be lost, and the capacity for successful interaction may be impaired. Intervention based on this frame of reference seeks to help the client to replace these developmentally acquired, but now lost, skills by the use of alternative strategies or man-made aids to daily living.

Earlier in this chapter, we reflected that theories of human development tend to focus on one aspect of development and that 'norms' are suggested for physical development, cognitive development and psychosocial development. In these terms, development is described as 'stage-like', each stage building on those previously attained. However, researchers also recognise that human development is holistic and integrated, each facet influencing the others, and that the maturation process suggests that genetic influences make possible steady developmental progess. This progress may be adversely affected, therefore, by the failure of genetic factors, as well as through non-supportive environmental experiences. Table 4.3 presents theories of normal development in terms of sensorimotor development, cognitive development, psychosocial development and the development of play.

Holistic nature of development

The six frames of reference for the practice of occupational therapy shown in Figure 4.2 will now be examined more closely. These, it has been suggested, protect the 'hard core' of our profession. All of these frames of reference view human development as an integrated whole. None is solely concerned with sensorimotor development, cognitive development or psychosocial development. All address the holistic nature of development and each seeks that clients may learn to function as 'whole' persons. It will be seen from

Table 4.3 Developmental Theories

Age (years)	Sensorimotor	Cognitive Piaget	Psychosocial Freud	Psychosocial Erikson	Play Parten	Play Piaget
0–1	Sits unsupported	Sensorimotor	Oral	Trust v. mistrust	Unoccupied play behaviour	Practice games
1–2	Reaches in all directions					
2–3			Anal	Autonomy v. shame	Onlooker play	
3–4						
4–5	Toilets in adult fashion		Phallic	Initiative v. guilt		
5–6	Dresses and undresses (child clothes)	Pre-operational			Solitary independent play / Parallel play	Symbolic games
6–7	Eats in adult fashion					
7–8	Hygiene care in adult fashion		Latency	Industry v. inferiority	Associative play	
8–9	Tie bow at back					
9–10	Tie neck tie					
10–11		Concrete operations			Cooperative play	
11–12						
12–18	Adult Hygiene care			Identity v. Role diffusion		Games with Rules
18–young Adult				Intimacy v. isolation		
Middle age		Formal operations	Genital	Generativity v. stagnation		
Ageing				Ego-integrity v. despair		

Table 4.3 that at about the chronological age of 12, the normally developing individual will have mastered the tasks needed for self-care, reading, writing, verbal communication, riding a bicycle and even (leaving aside the issue of legal constraints) driving a car. He will have mastered the skills necessary for the practical aspects of work – the ability to follow instructions, to judge when a task is completed to a required standard, and to stay with a task until it is completed, all of which remain within the cognitive realm of concrete operations.

Stages and crises of normal development

Concurrently, the normally developing individual will have addressed the stages of psychosocial development identified by Freud, and the crises which Erikson sees as conflicts between the self and society which, when successfully resolved, equip the individual with trusting expectations, a sense of self-control and the capacity for initiative.

From Table 4.3, it may be seen that the first such crisis, resulting in either trust or mistrust, occurs during the time-frame identified by Freud as the oral stage of development – the time when the infant's gratification is sought through sucking and chewing, and when expectations of receiving this gratification will engender an attitude of trust in a society which provides this gratification.

The crisis resulting in either autonomy or shame occurs during the time identified by Freud as the stage of anal gratification – the time during which early toilet training may enhance autonomy, engendering the beginnings of pleasure in self-control and early decision making, or result in shame as the result of society's scorn or punishment.

The time between 3 and 6 years of age is categorised by Freud as the phallic stage of development, during which the Oedipus or Electra complex is addressed and hopefully resolved. This is also the time for the emergence of the 'superego', the internalised monitor of values. Kohlberg suggests that until about 10 years of age, the child's moral reasoning emphasises the external control of others; from this time onwards, however, the child begins to internalise some of the moral standards of others who are deemed to be significant. The struggle to resolve the Oedipus/Electra complex and to establish a gender identity coincides with the crisis Erikson identifies as a conflict of guilt versus initiative – initiative developed by trust and autonomy and required for the beginnings of a socially acceptable sense of 'self', versus guilt resulting from a failure to do so.

From about 6 to 12 years of age is, according to Freud, the 'latency' stage, during which, he suggests, a diffusion of libidinal energy occurs. This, too, is the time wherein Erikson sees conflict arising around industry versus inferiority – often experienced through the challenge of school achievement and social interaction.

Successfully resolved, the life crises thus far encountered enable the adolescent to experience a feeling of self-worth, and to enter early adulthood with the tools necessary to establish an identity. Failure in the resolution of these early challenges results in a confused and diffused role, one with no clear commitment to any adult life goals.

Implications for practice

Those occupational therapists who work primarily with clients in a psychiatric setting will be accustomed to the medical diagnoses of schizophrenia, acute anxiety, depression or obsessive compulsion. However, the symptoms with which such clients present may be identified as poor concentration, unwillingness to take risks in decision making, isolation or a distorted perception of reality. All the evidence of mistrust, or shame and guilt, or inferiority, and almost certainly of an unclear identity may exist. In fact, it could be suggested that the establishment of an identity satisfactory to the client is always the hoped-for outcome of intervention. This identity may be different from the one the client had striven so hard for before disease or trauma made necessary the slow and often painful development and acceptance that another is now needed; or be an identity the client will come to develop through the process of 'recapitulation', the going back over, the second chance to try to resolve the crises of psychosocial development.

The frame of reference based on general systems theory focuses specifically on developmentally acquired deficiencies in role performance and on the distress experienced by individuals whose roles are diffused and inappropriate – the developmental inadequacy and the faulty resolution of earlier crises leading to inadequate understanding and performance of the roles which are normally a potential by the age of 12. It would seem, then, that development beyond the chronological age of about 12 years is concerned with an extension of sensorimotor skills, an application of cognitive abilities, an ability to enlarge and more firmly establish a personal identity and a recognition of the part played by 'rules' governing behaviour within a given society, which, in itself, determines the need for changing roles.

The practice of occupational therapy could, then, be said to address faulty development in the areas normally integrated by the age of 12. This is not to suggest that our clients' 'real' age is limited to 12 years, rather that our practice focuses on developmental tasks normally mastered by about that age, whether our practice is concerned with prevention, intervention, rehabilitation or maintenance. This perception of occupational therapy practice will be examined again at a later stage. However, the next few chapters focus on further areas of knowledge from which practice is derived (e.g. areas relating to change, learning and skill), and activity as the means by which we practise.

5. Concepts of occupational therapy: learning and skill acquisition

Learning continues to influence development throughout the whole of the human lifespan. Although most health professionals are interested in the learning process in this general sense, *specific* learning principles are of concern to occupational therapists, who aim chiefly to help clients acquire competent forms of behaviour through activity-based intervention. Moreover, occupational therapists envisage the learning process as one that can be planned, promoted and evaluated in line with treatment goals and established principles.

LEARNING THEORY: THE FORMATION OF HABITS

We know that learning has occurred whenever a change is evident in the organism that cannot be explained by instinct or maturation. This change occurs when the organism interacts with the environment and, in humans, may take the form of a new way of thinking or some new behaviour or approach to problem-solving. Sometimes the change is beneficial and adaptive, but this is not always so. People often and heedlessly build up a repertoire of incompetent habits, such as may relate, for example, to poor time management, work behaviour or social skills

James and Meyer

The first notable psychologist to write on the role of habit in everyday life was William James (1842–1910), brother of Henry, the novelist, and a gifted writer of prose in his own right. In his *Principles of Psychology*, published in 1890 after 12 years of preparation, James observed that it is habit that ties people to their given life roles, and that is largely responsible for preventing social rebellion. He also offered advice on the cultivation of useful habits, suggesting that we first make firm resolutions, then never allow an exception to planned behaviour until the new set of habits is firmly rooted. Although James recognised the central role of habit in human behaviour, he never adhered to what later became known as the behaviourist perspective. He was always deeply interested in free will and consciousness in human nature, and never subscribed to the view that learning is only and always a physiological process, or that it is the sole determinant of behaviour.

James' holistic perspective was shared by the influential psychiatrist Adolf Meyer (1866–1950). Meyer (1917) objected to prevailing diagnostic categories and argued that mental disorders are best conceived of as faulty habits of daily living. These can only be understood, he claimed, in the context of the total personality, and in the light of the many interacting factors that conspire to bring them about. Meyer's *psychobiology* remained an important influence until its inherent eclecticism became unfashionable with the rise of behaviourism.

Classical conditioning: Watson and Pavlov

While recognising learning and habit formation as important aspects of development, Meyer and James were never materialist and certainly never tried to explain human beings in terms of learned habits alone. It fell to J. B. Watson (1878–1958) to introduce this particular form of reductionism. Watson was a pragmatic, down-to-earth investigator, who grew weary of contemporary psychology's concern with introspection and its attendant philosophical problems. He ruled a study of mind out of court, claimed that a science of behaviour should focus only on observables, and persuaded his followers that the investigation of stimulus-response connections was the key to understanding organisms. His most notable publications appeared during the 1910s and, in due course, these received considerable support from the experiments of Ivan Pavlov (1849–1936) in Russia, on the digestive system in dogs. This happy coincidence (we can hardly say 'meeting of minds') led to the prevailing belief that learning is nothing more or less than classical conditioning, and that behaviour is grounded in conditioned reflexes. A key idea in Pavlov's work is that the organism (e.g. a dog) can learn to respond to a conditioned stimulus (e.g. a buzzer) in the same way as it would naturally respond to an unconditioned one (e.g. meat powder), provided that the stimuli are presented closely together in time (i.e. are contiguous). Training by classical conditioning requires frequent pairing of stimuli and, in instances such as that of Pavlov's dogs, the principle of *contiguity* is central, as is the concept of *associative learning* (that is, learning a similar response to two or more stimuli). These and other principles, such as that of *extinction* (see below), also form part of the vocabulary of an even more influential behavioural theory of learning, that of B. F. Skinner.

Box 5.1 Skinner's theory of operant conditioning

In classical conditioning, a reflex-like response is elicited by a stimulus, and the paired stimulus precedes the response, no matter what the organism does. In operant conditioning, it is the consequences of an action that determine whether it is likely to be repeated. In '*The Behaviour of Organisms*' (1938) and subsequent publications, Skinner introduced the concept of an *operant*. An operant is Skinner's term for any emitted response that affects the environment. He wrote that operant behaviour is at first random as the organism (typically a rat or pigeon) spontaneously 'operates' on its environment. Skinner's theory hinges on the concept of *reinforcement*. If some behaviour produces a desirable result (positive reinforcement), it is repeated, whereas if the outcome is painful or otherwise undesirable (negative reinforcement), the organism learns to behave in some way that terminates the aversive stimulus. Skinner also distinguishes between primary and secondary reinforcement. A primary reinforcer (e.g. food) is one that increases the likelihood of a response of its own accord, whereas the reward value of a secondary reinforcer has to be learned by association. Money, praise and token rewards for achieving objectives are common secondary positive reinforcers. Reinforcement delivered immediately after a response is more effective than delayed reinforcement.

   When an instructor is attempting to direct and control an organism's behaviour, she may at first reinforce responses that only approximate to the desired one, then only those that approach more closely the target behaviour. This procedure is known as 'shaping.' Again, where every approximate response is initially reinforced, the learner is said to be on a 'schedule of continuous reinforcement'. While this schedule is useful early in training, it is neither practical nor fully effective as a long-term strategy. To maintain improved performance, the instructor now uses 'partial reinforcement', in which only a proportion of correct or target responses are rewarded. Partial reinforcement is highly effective. Laboratory animals trained in this way show high frequencies of response, and often continue to respond enthusiastically after reinforcement is withdrawn. Withholding reinforcement for a long period, however, gradually leads to extinction of the conditioned behaviour. When this happens the animal or person's pattern of response returns to the pretraining base level, although the conditioned behaviour may reappear after rest in a process known as 'spontaneous recovery'. This occurs in the absence of renewed reinforcement, and demonstrates that the trained animal differs from its untrained counterpart. However. response strength in spontaneous recovery is generally less than that present before extinction occurred.

Applications of operant conditioning

Skinner's central tenet is that behaviour is governed by its consequences. His theory is a variation on traditional habit-formation theory, in that the association established is between behaviour and its results instead of between two stimuli, as is the case in classical conditioning. Where the principles of behavioural learning have been applied to humans*, classical conditioning has been the preferred method for training autonomic responses, while operant methods were deemed best for teaching global, skeletal types of behaviour. Classical conditioning has, therefore, been the method of choice for modifying undesirable emotional reactions, and its widest application has been in desensitising phobias according to procedures advocated by Wolpe (1958). More recently, however, it

---

* Sackett & Fitzgerald (1983) provides a useful introduction to behaviour therapy, and includes several concepts which cannot be treated fully in the present text.

has been found that operant conditioning can be equally effective in modifying responses mediated by the autonomic nervous system. For example, subjects can learn to control heart rate and blood pressure when reinforcement is provided as biofeedback.

Token economies Despite the above findings, the impact of operant conditioning procedures remains greatest when implemented in an institutional setting. The classical experiments in this area have been carried out by Ayllon and coworkers (e.g. Ayllon & Haughton 1962), and these have paved the way for a number of follow-up studies, typically involving psychiatric patients. One such study (Drovet 1983) is of particular interest because occupational therapy staff played an important part in setting up the behaviour modification programme in question. The programme, which was carried out at Horton Hospital, Epsom, was aimed at changing the behaviour of fairly long-term schizophrenic patients. It followed the conventional format, whereby some subjects received contingent token reinforcement, while others received some alternative form of treatment or reward. For those clients whose target behaviour was rewarded by tokens, reinforcement was contingent on participation in daily living activities, such as cookery, homecare, group activities, and also crafts and social skill programmes. Nurses also set targets relating to personal hygiene and socially acceptable behaviour, having first identified individual deficits and agreed as a team on priorities for modification. A check list was used to record reinforcement procedures and to monitor patient progress. Subjects included several individuals for whom no incentive to date had promoted cooperation. The authors of the report concluded that even these patients showed marked improvement following behavioural intervention.

Token economies are so called because tokens administered to reinforce targeted behaviour can be used by clients to 'buy' snacks, television viewing time, or whatever. The method can benefit staff as well as clients, since staff morale is increased upon witnessing the positive results of a programme in which they have participated. However, although token economies have produced remarkable improvement, their long-term value is open to question. Behaviours targeted for reinforcement tend to be highly specific, as are the criteria for their reinforcement, but this relationship is seldom maintained in a family or community setting. This discontinuity of reinforcement creates problems for patients who have completed a training programme and thereafter emerge to face the challenges of the outside world.

Reinforcement discontinuity The problem of reinforcement discontinuity is not limited to token economies. An example is provided by studies aimed at modifying the drinking behaviour of alcoholics. Some years ago, Californian psychologists set up a regime in which subjects had their drinking patterns monitored by video and received negative reinforcement (mild electric shocks) whenever they drank too much or too fast (Sobell & Sobell 1976). The programme directors took the view that alcoholic drinking reflects a maladaptive habit, not a disease, and their treatment goal was controlled imbibing in place of abstinence. They reported that two years after the original programme, subjects trained in this way were more in control of their drinking than a comparable group who had been taught to abstain. However, studies conducted a few years later by other researchers cast doubt on this claim. When the original sample was tracked down, it was discovered that many had not been honest in the follow-up interview (Pendery et al 1982). Within a year of behavioural treatment, two-thirds of the sample had required admission to hospital and several subsequently died of alcohol-related problems. While subjects had been motivated towards controlled social drinking, 'we couldn't', as one put it, 'find a bar with electric shocks'.

Training programmes such as the above, which lean heavily on aversive conditioning, are not recommended by Skinner. He advocates the use of positive rather than negative reinforcement, principally on grounds of its greater effectiveness. Certainly, of all the various conditioning principles, it is those relating to positive reinforcement that are of greatest use to the occupational therapist in her work. Yet even when teaching a craft or skill, the therapist will need to draw on other principles as well. Conditioning principles *are* relevant to the teaching process, but so too are principles relating to cognition and motivation which are outside the behaviourist frame of reference. Moreover, behaviourist philosophy (as a *global* philosophy) is not compatible with the humanistic perspective espoused by occupational therapy.

Skinner's philosophy

Skinner has been called a radical behaviourist because he rejects psychological and even physiological explanations of what we do, and accepts the environment alone as a determinant of behaviour. His position is atheoretical, in that he eschews conventional explanations in favour of *descriptions* of responses, together with the observable conditions or contingencies that are most likely to bring them about. In *Beyond Freedom and Dignity* (1972) Skinner has provided a non-technical behavioural analysis of culture and humankind. He reiterates his contention that all our behaviour is conditioned, and that what we think or feel has no bearing on it. He argues forcibly that humans are not free, although admittedly we like to cling to the illusory notions of freedom and choice. And because we are not free, we are not accountable for our actions, so that the whole concept of personal responsibility is a myth.

Critique

Naturally, cognitive psychologists and philosophers of rationalist persuasion object to a philosophy so much at odds with their own. In particular, Skinner's determinism and the allied passivity inherent in his view of man has come under attack. It can further be argued that his view of science is mistaken, in that he equates progress with methodology (which he rightly insists should be rigorous), while neglecting the role of theory. If Skinner's arguments are carried to their logical conclusion, theories are no more than conditioned responses, and were this indeed the case it is difficult to see how science could ever have advanced. Skinner has argued, too, that all our statements are also learned responses, and it was this denial of creativity in language that drew cogent and influential criticism from the linguist, Noam Chomsky.

Chomsky's criticisms In *Verbal Behaviour* (1957) Skinner argued that language is learned by the association of words and corresponding stimuli (a 'tact' relationship) and by reinforcement. When reinforcement follows a request (or 'mand') the words used are likely to be repeated in similar situations. Verbal behaviour is related to stimuli in several other ways, but the relationship is always one in which stimuli *control* what is said.

Chomsky (1959) attacked this account in a notoriously scathing review. He argued that far from being controlled by stimuli, the creativity of language is one of its most obvious characteristics. Human speech is not limited to utterances heard or reinforced in the past. People are quite capable of constructing novel sentences (witness the sentences that make up this book), and frequently do so. They are likewise capable of understanding other people's novel utterances.

Chomsky's own theoretical position is that, instead of learning an endless series of stimulus-response connections, children in fact acquire a working knowledge of the rules governing language. They then use these rules to generate new sentences. He proposes that children are biologically predisposed to construct a grammar, following exposure to a linguistic environment which is typically imperfect. This predisposition accounts for the speed of language acquisition in the early years and for its regular course of development across cultures.

Chomsky's theory provides a better explanation of language development than does Skinner's. Firstly, it would take several decades of exposure, if not a life-time, to build up the stimulus-response chains that are claimed in behaviourist theory to underlie language. Secondly, Skinner's theory cannot account for novel utterances, particularly the generation of embedded sentences – sentences in which two or more simple sentences are transformed into a more complex one. Thus, 'The gods like some people.' and 'Those people die young.' would become 'Those whom the gods love die young.' We frequently use sentences of this type and there is no limit to the number of embedded sentences that can be constructed in any language. They are not merely imitative and cannot therefore be explained by reinforcement. Developmental psycholinguistics has shown that even very young children construct utterances for which they have not been reinforced. When they form such plurals as 'mouses' or 'foots', or when they say, 'I goed' or 'I runned', they are clearly overextending a rule they have acquired, and are not merely imitating adult speech. Again, it is unlikely that 'creative mistakes' such as 'allgone hot' can be explained by imitation or reinforcement.

Conditioning versus cognitive principles Although Chomsky's criticism focused on Skinner's account of language, it succeeded in drawing attention to weaknesses in behaviourism on a wider scale. While undoubtedly much of our behaviour is learned, conditioning principles cannot account for the totality of it, and Chomsky's insistence on human rationality prompted a revival of interest in cognitive principles. In addition to traditionally influential cognitive theory, such as that of Piaget or Gestalt insight learning, there was renewed interest in the concept of the person as a scientist. This conceptualisation, introduced by Kelly (1955), holds that each of us develops a theory about the world in which we live in order to understand it better. Our theories take the form of organised personal constructs, which provide us with a framework for making sense of our circumstances. We are not, then, dehumanised and passive responders to stimuli, rather we respond to events in terms of how we construe them.

Fransella (1982) has observed that 'above all else, the occupational therapist is a teacher'. This being so, the therapist will need to be informed of the variety of learning principles that prevail, and must be able to decide when conditioning principles apply and when cognitive principles are more relevant. For example, when the therapist is teaching some craft or skill, providing an explanation of the task's relevance and therapeutic purpose (i.e. applying cognitive principles) is clearly worthwhile. Conditioning techniques – in particular, the provision of positive reinforcement – are relevant to inducing smooth performance, yet, even at this stage of skill learning, there will be individual differences in how reinforcement and the goals of intervention are perceived. As Fransella points out, some individuals might take the view that a particular task is a waste of time, or that it involves unnecessary discomfort. Others may see its accomplishment as a positive step on the road to recovery. Obviously, then, it is vitally important for the therapist to understand that there are individual differences in how the objectives of skill teaching are evaluated. Nowadays, in view of the limitations of radical behaviourism, the more influential theories of skill learning acknowledge that conditioning and cognitive principles play an equally important part in the acquisition process.

HUMAN SKILLS

During their lives, humans master an astonishing array of skills. Mastery begins in infancy, with the emergence of hand-eye co-ordination, and continues, albeit at a slower pace, in the later years. Most skills are adaptive or oriented to enjoyment. Many are culture-specific, but all societies require skills of some sort from their members, and these change as cultures evolve. Primitive cultures emphasise the skills that benefit survival, and even in the Stone Age, man had an impressive range of these. They had to know how to hunt and trap their prey, how to create fire, how to roast meat, make clubs from wood and sew animal skins together for clothing. More advanced societies tend to favour a division of labour and specialised skills.

Occupational therapists teach two broad classes of skill: *motor* (or perceptual-motor) skills and *social/communicative* skills. The focus in this chapter will be on motor skills, since a great deal of professional practice is geared to facilitating these. Moreover, since occupational therapy is principally concerned with eliciting competent behaviour in self-care, productivity and leisure, the principles which underlie skill acquisition in these areas merit a thorough discussion.

The nature of skill

We acquire skills in order that we may adapt efficiently and effectively to the circumstances of our lives. Skills are therefore goal-directed or, as Lovell (1982) puts it, 'are intended to achieve a predictable result with the maximum certainty of success and minimum expenditure of time and effort'. Skilled performance further involves the organisation of component activities into a sequence, in which one action typically serves as a cue for another. Thus, Fitts (1964) has defined a skilled response as 'one in which receptor-effector-feedback processes are highly organized, both spatially and temporarily'. The basic physiological aspect of the process is that receptors detect incoming sensory information and prompt appropriate effector responses in the form of muscle movements. But this is by no means the whole story (Fig. 5.1). Between sensory input and muscular output, there is always the issue of deciding what information should be acted upon, and what ignored. Skilled performance thus has a psychological dimension, in addition to a physical one, in which memory, perception and

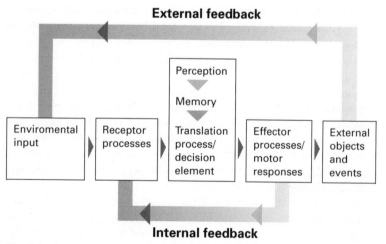

Fig. 5.1 A model of the constituent factors in skilled sensorimotor performance.

decision-making elements are involved. These mediating elements are said to make up the translation process inherent in skill. Feedback is also an important element, and denotes the process whereby information we receive as a result of our own performance, is then used to modify our subsequent efforts. Sometimes, feedback comes from our successes and failures at a task, at other times from our instructor; but just as frequently it comes from our internal kinesthetic sense, which yields sensory information about the smoothness, accuracy and suitability of the actions we have performed. Physiologically, the kinesthetic sense is a highly important aspect of skill, and Lovell (1982) observes that without it none of the carefully controlled physical movements that characterise the process would be possible.

Skills versus habits

Because skills are learned, they were for many years thought of as being more or less identical with habits, and it was believed that complex skills were acquired by chaining simple habits together. Conditioning techniques therefore dominated approaches to training, and were particularly popular during World War II, in view of the twin needs to train soldiers and retrain civilians in a variety of practical occupations.

Skinnerian techniques and the habit model of skill were finally challenged only some years after the war had ended. Oldfield (1959), for example, observed that a habit is a stereotyped response which, as learning progresses, becomes increasingly independent of its environment. A skill, on the other hand, is modified by the situation in which it occurs, and by other forms of feedback. Above all, the skilled performer has learned to respond *appropriately*, not rigidly, to external events.

Current perspectives on skill also take the view that information regarding performance is not merely a form of reinforcement. Operant teaching procedures are based on the principle that reinforcement, if it is to be effective, must follow the execution of a response. However, information in the form of guidance can be equally effective when provided concurrently or in advance of training. Stammers & Patrick (1975) point out that guidance has been termed 'error-free' training, because it eliminates mistakes and thereby prevents the learner from repeating errors that must subsequently be unlearned – a process that frequently occurs when trainees make errors early in the learning process. A comprehensive perspective on skill must take cognitive elements into account, and must acknowledge the fact that the learner requires information if he is to understand the task and its goals in the first place – a facet of skill that is overlooked in behaviourist theory.

Kielhofner (1985) has drawn attention to a further important psychological dimension to skill acquisition, namely that of belief. If a person is to master a given set of skills, he must believe that they are relevant and useful, and that he can acquire them success-fully with appropriate effort. Of course, success depends on having a realistic picture of one's own ability. Kielhofner & Burke (1985) point out that people with disability often have a distorted view of their skills and potential. This may be due to the impact of trauma and disease, or may arise from restricted learning opportunities or attempts to perform beyond one's capacity.

Evidently, teachers of skill need to have a large repertoire of con-cepts available as guides, since the range of human skills is wide, and principles applicable to simple tasks can seldom account ade-quately for complex learning. For these reasons, research over recent decades has stressed cognitive factors in addition to those which pertain to habit. Two approaches in this tradition remain highly influential. One is that of Fitts and his coworkers (Fitts & Posner 1967) who have identified phases of motor skill acquisition; the second is the information processing model of skilled behaviour to which a number of investigators have contributed.

Phases of motor skill aquisition

On the basis of his work with pilots and professional sports instruc-tors, Fitts proposed that skills are acquired in three stages: the *cognitive, associative* and *autonomous stages*.

Cognitive stage

The initial, cognitive phase is characterised by discussion between trainee and instructor which helps to elucidate what is required and identify errors to be expected. The learner may in fact begin to attempt some aspects of the task but, as he does so, the instructor draws attention to flaws in these attempts that might otherwise be overlooked. Guidance of this kind can be more effective than rein-forcement alone (Stammers & Patrick 1975), and management of this phase by the instructor can reduce learning time considerably.

Associative stage

The associative stage is that of error elimination and the formation of new habits. It is at this time that Skinnerian principles most clearly apply. At the outset, the learner's behaviour remains influenced by previously established habits. If these are compatible with the novel skill, positive transfer of training is likely to occur. Negative transfer obtains when the responses required are in opposition to a set already learned in a similar situation. In this circumstance, the rate of learning a new skill is impaired. The duration of the second stage, in which correct responses become 'fixed' with practice, depends on the task's complexity. Fitts & Posner (1967) report that, for trainee aircraft pilots, the instruction time required to reduce the risk of serious error is typically 10 hours.

Autonomous stage

Although there is a degree of overlap between the successive stages proposed by Fitts, the associative and autonomous stages can be distinguished in terms of the fluency, accuracy and speed that characterise skill in the latter phase. In this autonomous stage, less processing is required, and the individual becomes resistant to distraction and stress. There is a fair amount of evidence that progress in skill does not cease once the autonomous phase is reached. Crossman (1959), for example, using speed of performance as an index of improvement, conducted a field study of workers engaged in making cigars on a hand-operated machine. He found that performance speed increased linearly over a 4-year span before it levelled off.

Concepts from information-processing theory

As discussed earlier in this chapter, skill acquisition is grounded in a receptor-effector process and in addition, involves a decision-making dimension intervening between stimulus and appropriate reactions. The nature and role of this cognitive dimension has preoccupied information theorists since the inauguration of this field of inquiry shortly after the last war. Early writers on the topic include Wiener (1948), who introduced the variant known as 'cybernetics' and Shannon (1948), who defined many of the field's basic concepts. These workers and their followers have found it useful to draw an analogy between human mental processes and the processing strategies of the computer. Information theorists are concerned with how the human operator's 'hardware' (brain and nervous system) and available 'software' (rules, motives, plans and programmes) equip him to receive and translate input which is then transformed into observable output.

According to information theory, input and information are not necessarily synonymous. Some types of input convey zero information because they contain nothing that reduces uncertainty. For example (Fitts & Posner 1967), an input statement to the effect that a coin flip is 'either heads or tails' does not constitute information: it does not reduce any doubts we might have about the outcome. On the other hand, a statement describing the direction of the coin's fall does count as genuine information. Since information reduces uncertainty, it naturally follows that the more an event decreases uncertainty, the greater is the amount of information that it transmits. It is, of course, possible to describe the relationship between statements and their information content mathematically. Shannon (1948) developed a host of mathematical theorems to express possible relationships, but these need not concern us here.

Information theory focuses on the fact that while our senses are constantly being bombarded by stimulation, we nevertheless develop a capacity in the course of skill acquisition to recognise, filter and organise only those signals that are relevant to the desired outcome (Fig. 5.2). Attention and perception are key concepts in the theory, and bear upon our responses to initial, task-related input and to feedback. Feedback may take the form of kinesthetic signals resulting from our own body movements, or it may come from the environment. Such non-kinesthetic feedback occurs, for example, when we compare our performance against some criterion, or respond to some comment by the instructor. Either way, feedback gives us information about the progress we are making and helps us to modify our activity. A further key notion in information theory is that the human operator has limited channel capacity: in other words, there are limits to our capacity to store, retrieve, code and analyse information, and any one set of signals must be cleared before others can be dealt with.

Trainee changes during skill acquisition

According to information processing theory, perception and reaction time are major processes affected by training. During the early stages of skill learning, perception is poorly organised. Trainees give indiscriminate attention to incoming signals, failing to recog-

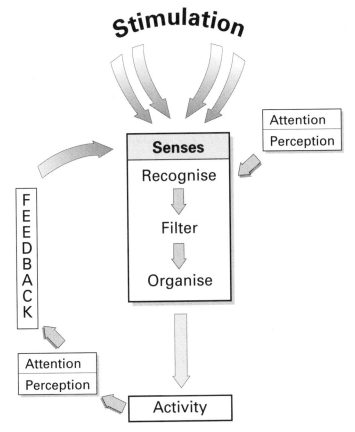

Fig. 5.2   Information theory.

nise that some of these yield no useful information and are thus
redundant. Gradually, scanning ability improves. The trainee
focuses on relevant signals alone, and becomes more efficient at
predicting their sequence. He becomes better, too, at sifting information for storage – an important gain in view of his limited
channel capacity. Task-related abilities are seen to change in the
contribution they make as the student progresses. For example,
Fleishman & Hempel (1955) found that when students were learning a discrimination reaction-time task over 15 trials, spatial ability
initially contributed 36% to performance, but only 11% at the end.
In general, once discriminative abilities improve, other features of
the task assume greater importance, and more time is available to
prepare for action.

Information theorists have traditionally used the concept of reaction time as a criterion of skill. Early investigators assumed that, as learning progresses, the interval between stimulus and response always becomes shorter. However, there are flaws in this line of argument. Principally, it overlooks the fact that responses must be not only quick, but also appropriate. The skilled performer often decides to delay some response in order to maximise appropriateness, and the trainee must likewise learn to anticipate events and time responses. As training progresses, discrimination and timing improve. The interval between signal input and response decreases – in other words, there is a decrease in *choice reaction time*. The concept of choice reaction time (as opposed to simple reaction time) is especially relevant to complex skills. Whereas learning a simple task typically involves few stimuli and a restricted set of responses, the performer of a more complex task is faced with a more complicated stimulus array. In this case, the performer must be able to make a choice as to what should be done in the presence of several stimuli, so that choice reaction time will clearly be longer, the more signals that are involved. Hick's (1952) law states that choice reaction time increases at a constant logarithmic rate as the amount of information conveyed by stimuli increases. The law holds true for people learning a wide variety of skills. However, as subjects become very skilled, choice reaction time remains constant even when additional information is being received.

Limitations on skill learning

There are several aspects of the task to be learned that may adversely affect performance. Indeed, many such factors reduce performance even in people who are already skilled.

Sensory overload

Possibly the most important factor is sensory overload which occurs when the trainee or skilled operator is presented with more information than he or she can adequately process. Performance in these circumstances declines, since, in information theory terms, the human 'channel capacity' is limited. Typically, the affected person ignores some signals that may be important, or makes processing errors that affect output. Another adjustment procedure is to delay responding in the short-term, then try to make good this delay at a time when input is less. Overload also reduces response precision (Miller 1960).

Sensory underload

Performance can likewise be diminished by sensory underload. This occurs when information input is excessively low to the extent that the task is perceived as boring. Vigilance tasks which require subjects to track infrequent or indistinct signals reveal the effects of underload. Vigilance tends to be adequate at the outset, then detection rates fall off. In general, tasks which are repetitive or set in monotonous surroundings reduce efficiency, since the ascending reticular formation system is not sufficiently aroused to maintain alertness.

Fatigue

Fatigue is another limiting factor. Because subjective reports are unreliable, and because fatigue itself is heavily influenced by motivation, researchers in this area tend to focus on performance changes over relatively prolonged periods. Welford (1968) notes that for the term 'mental fatigue' to have any real meaning, these performance changes should involve a degree of impairment in capacity or sensitivity which must be reversible following rest. He has isolated four main types of fatigue-induced change. Firstly, there are sensory or perceptual changes in which sensitivity and visual acuity are reduced and, secondly, sensorimotor performance slows down. Subjects whose speed of performance is reduced by tiredness tend to neglect important signals or omit required actions. Performance gradually suffers a disruption as they try to make amends for these omissions, only to lose further time in the process. Under these conditions, subjects typically show bursts of overactivity, coupled with anxiety. A third effect is that timing becomes irregular as subjects become distracted and attend to irrelevant signals. Fourthly, there may be disorganisation of performance.

Massed versus distributed training

While it is unlikely that patients in occupational therapy will undertake tasks that tire them unduly, there remains the question of how much time should be spent learning a particular activity (massed versus distributed training). The short answer is that it depends on the task. Concentrating practice over unbroken or 'massed' periods can be more effective for verbal learning. However, the material is likely to be forgotten soon afterwards, as those

Box 5.2

Welford (1968) discusses disorganisation with reference to the classical Cambridge experiments in which pilots with brief wartime training were studied as they adjusted to flying conditions in a simulated cockpit. Subjects were assessed over 2-hour intervals, under simulated heavy cloud circumstances. The results, as reported by Bartlett (1943), showed that fatigued pilots often made correct responses in the wrong order, revealing a breakdown in capacity to coordinate the task as a whole. Judgement was also impaired in that, as standards declined, pilots actually thought they were performing more efficiently.

who cram for examinations have discovered. Distributed practice – in which rest pauses occur between training sessions – is generally thought to be more effective in the longer term. It is undoubtedly a better approach to activity learning, and induces less fatigue than massed training. However, some thought should be given to the issue of rest periods: if they are not appropriately timed, forgetting may occur.

Form of disability

Thus far, the limitations on learning outlined have highlighted task-related and learning variables that have general application. However, individualistic variables must also be taken into account, and there are as many of these as there are forms of disability. Shingledecker (1981) has pointed out that while the acute break-down of skill produced by task demands and similar stressors can be alleviated by improving task conditions, chronic breakdown due to handicap is less easily remedied. Although technology has inspired the development of prosthetic and orthotic devices, and many sensory aids, these are often designed without due regard for the human operator. Shingledecker proposes that the information-processing model might be of benefit to designers, because it specifies how sensory and motor deficits affect central mechanisms and, ultimately, performance. Studies of amputees (hand and/or arm) given a choice of methods to control a prosthesis, have shown that grasp and placing ability is better when the artificial limb is powered by electromyographic (EMG) potential than by pull switches, although this superiority diminishes in the case of higher level amputations. Nevertheless, subjects invariably prefer EMG control because it is less tiring and less ambiguous. Designers of these systems apparently fail to realise that control positions should be relatively easy to discriminate (the EMG method appears to be superior in this regard), and that having too many controls reduces both ease and speed of performance – an outcome which Shingledecker suggests is exactly as one would expect in view of the user's limited channel capacity and Hick's reaction time law.

TEACHING SKILLS

The process of teaching a skill can be guided by the general learning principles already outlined. However, some adaptations and additional principles are required. The first task of the instructor is that of analysing the skill in question, and deciding on this basis what method of teaching should be adopted. A basic decision concerns whether whole or part training is preferable. If the part method is used, the first subcomponent of the task is initially learned, then the second, and the sequence continues until finally the parts are combined and the task practised as a whole. There are other ways of combining part practice. For example, the student can learn subparts one and two individually, then combine these before progressing to the third part of the task. This variation is known as 'progressive part training'. Studies of the relative merits of these approaches have produced mixed results and it is clear from these that the nature of the task is of paramount importance in choosing the teaching method.

Naylor's review of the evidence (Naylor 1962, Blum & Naylor 1968) suggests that the first aspect of the skill to be taken into account is its level of *organisation* – the degree of inter-relatedness of components. If this is low then as the task increases in *complexity* – in terms of the demands placed on the learner – part methods become more effective. Under conditions of high organisation, whole methods are found to be more effective as task complexity increases.

Stammers & Patrick (1975) maintain that the degree of *interdependence* between elements should also be taken into account. This variable, highlighted by Annett & Kay (1956), is not quite the same as organisation, although it would seem to be so on the surface. The term in fact refers to whether or not the operator's responses influence subsequent signals. If they do so, the elements are interdependent, otherwise they are independent. Given that complexity influences the choice of teaching method (mainly as it increases), this extra dimension facilitates decisions concerning method when complexity is low. For example, if organisation and complexity are low, the whole method remains preferable if interdependence is also low; but under the same conditions, if interdependence is high, then the part training method becomes more appropriate.

Task analysis

Since, as Kielhofner (1985) observes, a skilled act is made up of subroutines that are organised into a hierarchy, these subroutines must be identified before training can proceed. Subroutines are organised units of movement which can, themselves, be broken down into component parts. This process of identifying the components of a skill, and charting their sequence is known as *task analysis*.

Definition of objectives

When an instructor or therapist is planning a teaching programme, she must, in the first place, define its objectives. These should be clearly stated at the outset and contain criteria for proficiency, preferably formulated in terms of observable performance. It is not sufficient to say what the student should 'understand' after training. Objectives must focus on what the student should be able to do. Information on the nature of the skill and the level of performance expected after training can be gleaned from several sources. Observing and interviewing experts at work, examining one's own experience, and using videotaped recordings are all useful techniques. Having gained an overall picture of the skill in question, the next step is to identify the subtasks involved and the order in which they occur.

The most straightforward approach is to take the first occurring element in a subroutine and use this as a starting point for further development. Decisions about what actually constitutes the first element are usually based on whether the preceding actions can typically be carried out without training. An example is given in Box 5.3 (see also Fig. 5.3).

Box 5.3   Teaching a tennis serve

A task analysis might usefully list baseline body position
(including details) as the first requirement for teaching.
Preceding actions, such as lifting the ball from the ground,
are unlikely to require training in normal circumstances.
The second subtask in the sequence concerns throwing up
the ball. Under this heading, a component task analysis
would typically describe the throwing action and list the
body adjustments that accompany the throw. The third
step in description would centre on how the ball is hit on
descent. The procedure continues until the subroutine is
analysed in full. Of course, the game of tennis involves
many subroutines other than serving, each of which is
analysed and taught before a synthesis can be achieved.

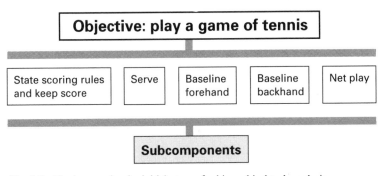

Fig. 5.3   Playing tennis: the initial stage of a hierarchical task analysis.

Another approach to task analysis is to descend hierarchically
from a global description of goals to that of constituent operations.
The starting point in this procedure, then, would not be the first
element in a subroutine but, rather, an outline of the overall objective, for example, 'play a game of tennis'. Analysis next centres
on operations at the next highest level, while at the third level, each
of these categories is analysed into suboperations. For each operation, rules of sequencing are stated, as are rules of selection if a
number of performance options are built into the task. To facilitate
teaching, the analyst also takes note of input and feedback cues that
prompt action. In line with the conventions of task analysis, an

operation is defined as a behavioural unit (Annett et al 1971) in order to avoid ambiguity. Specifying the operations and level of organisation involved in a task makes it easier for the instructor to decide on the most appropriate teaching method.

Assessment of outcome

Task analysis also facilitates assessment. It not only embodies a statement of expected performance at the end of training, but, since it specifies subtasks as well, also contains criteria for evaluating performance along the road to final mastery. There remains the issue of evaluating individual differences prior to training. The assessment of entering behaviour is particularly important where manipulative and psychomotor ability is impaired. Assessment at this level enables the instructor to decide whether the student requires special training to develop the prerequisite basic abilities, or whether the best course of action is to select a more suitable task.

Verbal and social skills

Various techniques exist to help people reproduce verbal material accurately. Chunking and imagery are popular methods of improving memory for telephone numbers, shopping lists and mathematical tables, but are of limited use where the material to be learned is complex. Investigators of verbal learning tend to explain the process in cognitive terms.

The cognitive approach

The cognitive approach originated in Gestalt psychology, which held that learning in general involves restructuring the perceptual field. The Gestalt school argued that learning occurs when the subject perceives a situation in a new way. Having reorganised the elements of a problem in such a way that a solution is facilitated, the learner who finally solves the problem does so by *insight*.

Wertheimer   The Gestalt psychologist, Wertheimer (1880–1943) was particularly interested in education. He believed that traditional teaching methods emphasised rote learning and mechanical application of rules at the expense of genuine understanding. In *Productive Thinking* (1945), he advocated flexible teaching methods aimed at encouraging insight-learning and creative problem-solving.

Ausubel   David Ausubel, like Wertheimer, is concerned with comprehension. He focuses on verbal learning and has outlined a set of principles which he recommends to teachers. Ausubel (1963) argues that simple laboratory-derived laws of learning have little relevance to academic material, as this kind of subject matter can only be mastered if it has meaning for the learner. He argues that meaning is a conscious experience in which concepts are organised within the cognitive structure in such a way that they are understood independently of a particular phrasing. They can therefore be expressed verbally in a number of ways without loss of meaning. His basic proposition is that new ideas can be meaningfully learned only to the extent that they can be related to already existing concepts.

Concerning instruction, Ausubel recommends that teaching new material should be preceded by a general introduction. The teacher who proceeds in this way is offering students a set of 'advance organisers' which will give a structure to learning. As teaching progresses, new subject matter should be presented clearly and should only expand on what is already known. However, the distinctive attributes of particular ideas must be emphasised to prevent forgetting. Ausubel's theory of meaningful verbal learning stresses that students should be called upon to express what they have learned in their own words, to discourage rote learning. Occupational therapists engaged in helping clients follow complex instructions will find Ausubel's principles useful, as will those who teach advanced skills requiring verbal explanation.

Social skills training

Social skills training focuses on both verbal and non-verbal components of social behaviour. It is widely used in institutional settings with those who have evident communication difficulties, and as a consumer service for clients who wish to become more confident in social interaction.

Prior to training, deficits in social behaviour are identified. Identification and analysis can be carried out by observing the client in a number of relevant situations, or by using interviews or questionnaires. Typically, the instructor sets training goals with reference to specific elements of social behaviour that appear to be flawed. At the non-verbal level, an individual may be using posture, facial expression, gesture and eye-contact inappropriately, or may be insensitive to the non-verbal signals of others. Aspects of verbal communication that may profit from training include tone of voice, greeting rituals and expressing oneself with confidence. Many people admit to difficulties in situations which require them to complain, refuse, apologise, issue instructions or make requests. Assertiveness training is geared to improving skills in these areas, and helps people to respond appropriately, rather than defensively or aggressively. A wide cross-section of people benefit from assertiveness training. Teachers, sales and managerial personnel find it useful, as do individuals who are trying to abstain from alcohol, drugs or nicotine. In the latter cases, trainees are taught to refuse proffered substances assertively, without anxiety. Social skills training programmes are widely used, too, with neurotic and psychotic individuals, with the aim of reducing social anxiety.

Methods Methods of social skills training include instruction, modelling, simple exercises, role-play and homework. Initially, the elements of verbal and non-verbal communication may be practised separately; later, they are integrated into a role-play scenario. Before beginning role-play, the skill in question is generally introduced and demonstrated by 'live' or filmed models. Trainees then act out the scenario themselves with other trainees, or with a partner from the training team. Feedback is supplied in the form of verbal comment by the trainer, comparison with the modelled performance or videotape-playback. Throughout the procedure, role-play is supplemented by reinforcement and guidance. Trainees are also encouraged to try out their newly acquired skills in the real world, and are given homework to practise between laboratory sessions.

Argyle (1969) has developed a social skills model which stresses motivation (see below). According to this model, all social behaviour is goal-directed, in the sense that when we interact with others we do so for a purpose, although we may not be fully aware of this. It may be that we wish to convey information, win the other person's approval or make a request. Whatever the reason, we are setting out to have some impact on the other person, and we may fail in this if we send out the wrong cues and do not reinforce the other's responses in the desired direction. Showing interest, smiling, nodding, listening and turn-taking are among the subtle processes that we use to modify another's behaviour and attain our goals. People who are successful at attaining their goals are said to have social competence, a competence which is itself the goal of social skills training.

Motivation

In attempting to explain why people behave as they do, behavioural scientists have frequently had recourse to the notion of motivation. Approaches to the problem vary. Some theorists equate motives with instincts or biological drives, and some with goal-seeking tendencies, while others differentiate between physiological and higher-order needs. Theorists have also differentiated between conscious and unconscious motives, learned and unlearned ones, and also between particular kinds of motivation, such as the need for achievement, all of which reflect individual differences. Some investigators of motivation prefer to draw up lists of motives deemed to underlie specific aspects of behaviour. However, this approach leaves a lot to be desired. To suggest that eating reflects hunger, or abasement an abasement motive, is to offer no valid explanation and, logically, involves circular reasoning.

Instead of identifying a plethora of individual motives, Hull (1943) concentrated on the common characteristics of motivation. He took a biological, neo-behaviourist view of motivation, which he conceptualised as one of several intervening variables between stimuli and responses. Focusing on the survival value of behaviour, he contended that motivation is grounded in the satisfaction of basic physiological needs. Animals, and especially humans, also have secondary needs, not essential for survival, but learned through association with primary ones. When an organism is deprived of something it needs, it is in a state of tension or 'drive'. The total drive state raises the body's level of activity, prompting the organism to seek ways of reducing the drive. Drive reduction is reinforcing, by analogy with the steady state principle of homeostasis, and responses which reduce drives are therefore rapidly learned. Hull's theory throws light on many behavioural phenomena. For example, it provides a framework in which to consider learned methods of reducing anxiety. People who find that alcohol and drugs are more effective than other means of reducing the drive state of anxiety are more likely to become dependent on them.

A problem with drive theory is that some motives have no biological basis, nor are they learned by association with a primary drive. Harlow's classical experiments with infant monkeys showed that the need for 'contact comfort' exists independently of the need for food (Harlow et al 1950). He also found that young monkeys have a natural tendency to explore the environment and find out how things work. Exploratory behaviour appears to reflect an underlying curiosity motive, for it does not depend on reinforcing some associated essential need.

One reason why so many theories prevail on the topic is that motivation cannot be observed directly. All we can ever see is behaviour, from which we infer the existence of motives. Probably the most popular current view of motivation is that of Maslow (Ch. 2). His classification of biological, social and higher-order needs has wide appeal, even for those who do not subscribe to his theory in its entirety.

Theories of motivation agree, at least implicitly, that living organisms tend to seek pleasure and avoid pain. Thus, at a non-biological level, being praised and approved of are generally pleasurable experiences which most people strive to attain. Likewise, the satisfaction of biological needs is intrinsically pleasurable, just as states of deprivation are unpleasant, prompting their reduction. Since the pleasure/pain principle applies to so many varieties of goal-directed behaviour, McClelland (1951) has defined a motive in broad terms as 'an expectancy of pleasantness or unpleasantness'. There remains the fact that even when goals are expected to bring about a pleasant experience (i.e. when they are perceived as incentives), individuals differ in the amount of energy they are prepared to expend in their pursuit. Again, any one individual may show variations in energy from situation to situation. Thus, De Cecco (1968, p 132) writes that 'motivation actually refers to those factors which increase and decrease the vigor of an individual's activity'.

The need for stimulation

While biological motives undoubtedly underpin a great deal of behaviour, they are hardly of central relevance to the behaviour of clients in an occupational therapy department. True, food (usually sweets) is sometimes used as a reward in therapy, and access to it has been made contingent on punctuality in some token economy programmes (e.g. Ayllon & Haughton 1962). Nevertheless, the concept of biological motivation is of limited value in relation to human learning, except to the extent that certain tasks and exercises may relate to pain-avoidance in the short or long term. Certainly, therapists are unlikely to deprive patients of food, water or sleep if their performance falls below expectations. As Maslow (1954) has pointed out, in circumstances where basic biological needs are met, they cease to function as powerful influences on behaviour.

The need for stimulation is not strictly a biological one, in that

Box 5.4   Heron's (1957) sensory-deprivation experiments

In a series of experiments, students were required to wear translucent goggles which admitted only homogenous light, and padding to reduce touch sensitivity. They were paid to lie alone on beds in a sound-proof room and tolerate these conditions for as long as possible (except for periods allotted to eating and basic needs.) Most students found that 8 hours of reduced stimulation was as much as they could take. Those who remained longer found it difficult to think clearly, and some began to hallucinate. The longer subjects chose to remain in the experiment, the more they became extremely restless and desperate for stimulus change. If given the chance to hear an out-of-date stock-market report, subjects would request that it be played repeatedly. Generally, disturbances induced by sensory deprivation lasted for some 24 hours after return to normal life.

an organism deprived of stimulation for a time will not die. Nevertheless, stimulation enhances physical well-being and is an important motivating factor in learning. Its importance for normal functioning is clear from a variety of studies carried out to assess the effects of sensory deprivation. Animals deprived of visual stimulation in early life show long-lasting perceptual deficits, suggesting atrophy of part of the visual system and, for humans, short-term deprivation is an unpleasant experience. In prisons, solitary confinement is one of the more severe forms of punishment administered, and researchers have found that subjects dislike taking part in sensory-deprivation experiments, even when paid well to do so (Box 5.4).

Social stimulation: Eric Berne

Eric Berne (1966) has observed that social conversation is often ritualistic and low in information content, yet valued at the same time for the stimulation it offers. The need for social stimulation, he argues, has its basis in the stimulus-hunger of infancy, which is satisfied by close contact with the mother to a degree that may never occur again. In the course of development, stimulus-hunger becomes partially transformed into recognition-hunger. This, in turn, is satisfied by contact with other people, which may take some physical form but which, more frequently, takes the form of symbolic 'stroking'.

Transactions

According to Berne, a 'stroke' is the fundamental unit of social action. Strokes include gestures of recognition – such as a nod of the head or a wave – and verbal ways of acknowledging another's presence. The process of exchanging a series of strokes is called a *transaction*. Berne argues that social stroking is biologically advantageous, and our need of it extremely powerful. Some individuals cannot manage transactions without antagonism, and even prefer the option of a likely quarrel to that of silence. Transactional analysis focuses on the games that incompatible people build into their relationship. It centres on the idea that, given our need for stroking, any form of social intercourse is deemed preferable to none at all.

Stimulation and learning

Stimulation arouses the nervous system and facilitates action. For learning purposes, moderate degrees of arousal, which may even be experienced as anxiety, are best for performance, although the optimal level of arousal depends on the difficulty of the task. A person in more likely to learn an activity that is stimulating in its own right, or presented in a stimulating way, than one which is subjectively judged to be boring. People are also more likely to learn activities that earn them social recognition and approval, either from their instructors or from peers in the training situation.

Activities which centre on arts, crafts and work-skills often have greater intrinsic interest than activities of a more routine nature. However, many disabled persons are unable to engage in these without first learning to use appropriate aids. Learning to manage supports, mouth-sticks, page turners and other aids can be uncomfortable and frustrating at the outset, as can the process of learning how to use specially adapted machinery and equipment for domestic or work purposes. In these circumstances, performance is more likely to be motivated by long-term goals. In addition to basic needs, humans have higher-order needs relating to independence, competence and self-esteem, and the instructor or therapist should keep in mind the task's potential for facilitating personal development.

Learning and higher-order needs

Theories which relate learning to higher-order needs, including self-actualisation, tend to be grounded in a general philosophy of human nature. Non-utilitarian philosophies of learning, which date back to Ancient Greece, typically emphasise intellectual and personal growth over pragmatic concerns, such as the acquisition of facts and specific abilities. The humanistic values inherent in the classical tradition waxed and waned in influence over the centuries, becoming most dominant during the Renaissance. Thereafter, their impact declined, although they have continued to influence educational systems to a greater or lesser degree. For example, Snygg & Combs (1959) have elaborated a personal development model in which they propose that education should help to realise each person's full potential at personal, social and intellectual levels. They relate learning to the need for self-esteem and self-acceptance, and argue that the main aim of education is self-enhancement.

Our outline of the values of occupational therapy (Ch. 3) makes it clear that the profession is grounded in humanistic values. Values concerning the client's self-directedness, personal responsibility, potential for self-enhancement and enhancement of health underlie professional practice. As Yerxa (1983) has pointed out, occupational therapists are concerned with strengthening the healthy aspects of individuals, and do not focus exclusively on pathology. However, there remains the possibility that the goals of a personal development model may appear too broad and remote in the context of the actual teaching situation. Instructors who are trying to help clients achieve stated objectives may prefer to think about these in terms of specified performance criteria and/or the more immediate value of the activity being taught. Mocellin (1984) has drawn attention to several 'vague and obscure' concepts that have found their way into the literature on occupational therapy in attempts to identify and develop a philosophical basis for practice. He is particularly critical of the terms 'coping' and 'adaptation' which have tended to replace fundamental concepts based on the therapeutic use of activities. Mocellin proposes instead (as noted earlier) that 'competence' and 'skills' should be core concepts in any acceptable theory of occupational therapy. He contends that the acquisition of skills promotes the experience of efficacy and control called competence; and that it is this experience, and not 'occupation', that is of therapeutic value.

Competence

It was Robert White (1959) who originally drew attention to the need for a concept such as competence to account for the tendency to strive for self-determination and control. He used the concept to denote the organism's capacity to interact *effectively* with its environment, thus emphasising the term's active – as opposed to respondent – connotations. White observed that even in childhood, exploratory play is geared towards achieving an effective familiarity with one's surroundings, and that in such play it is possible to discern a theme of mastery. In a thorough analysis of alternative explanations, he rejected drive deficit theory, claiming instead that man's persistent tendency to explore and control the environment reflects 'effectance' or competence motivation. The motive is characterised by an expectancy of efficacy, and it is this which prompts us to learn necessary skills. Competence has biological significance, since homeostatic mechanisms are limited in their powers of ensuring survival. For example, they are adequate in enabling us to adjust to mild fluctuations in outdoor temperature, but under conditions of marked variation, humans must learn to build dwelling places and construct heating and air-cooling systems. The motivation towards competence thus helps us defy the hazards of fate. In an interesting development of his theme, White suggested that the competence motive is not so strong as the primary biological drives. Were this the case, contingent behaviour would tend towards rigidity. The ability to deal adequately with situational demands requires flexibility and breadth of learning, which is best achieved when motivation is moderate. Strong motive strength accelerates and narrows learned behaviour, while moderate degrees favour steady, cumulative learning. Thus, many of the skills needed to transact effectively with the environment are acquired under conditions of leisurely exploration.

Mocellin notes that White (1971) has specifically related competence to the practice of occupational therapy, and points out that the term does not equate with excellence. Relating the concept to skill acquisition, he writes that education is the profession's major tool and that 'there is no difference between education and "treatment" in occupational therapy because, when the process is analysed what has been called therapy consists essentially of teaching, learning and of using residual skills and competencies' (Mocellin 1984, p 17).

Sutcliffe (1984) has observed that, in the course of training, occupational therapists are essentially educated for health (although too often actual techniques are slanted towards 'picking up the pieces'). She argues that the profession's focus on teaching life-skills and facilitating development reflects a curriculum that could benefit many individuals other than students of occupational therapy. Sutcliffe suggests that occupational therapy is really occupational education. Thus, like Mocellin, she views education as the profession's major tool.

This chapter has provided a relatively general analysis of the learning process, the coverage of specific skills having been kept to a minimum as a matter of policy. In the next two chapters, we return to the themes of skill acquisition and task analysis. However, the focus will now be on principles relating to activity, and on the role of activity and task mastery in occupational therapy.

6. The principles of occupational therapy

THE NATURE AND PURPOSE OF PRINCIPLES

In Chapter 1, it was stated that: 'the term principle embodies the concept of regularities. Principles are used to account for observed regularities of relationship. . .'. For example, the principle of reinforcement is a summary statement of the relationship between behaviour and its consequences; or Archimedes' principle – which most of us learn in school and which we see demonstrated almost every day – which concerns the observed regularity with which a solid will displace liquid into which it is placed. Potatoes placed in a saucepan of water cause the level of water to rise; when we get into a bath of water that water level rises, and so on. The significant factor about this, or any other principle, is that it is observed to occur with regularity.

The purpose of principles of practice, for occupational therapy or any profession, is two-fold: they (1) provide security to the practitioner and consistency to practice and thus (2) contribute significantly to the establishment and maintenance of a clear professional identity. As was also noted in Chapter 1, our profession has come up with numerous statements, each endeavouring to define occupational therapy, but our practice is still perceived as diffuse and lacking in consistency. The Commission set up by the College of Occupational Therapists in the late 1980s, with a brief to report on the existing and future role of occupational therapy in the United Kingdom, indicated the lack of a professional identity and suggested that this lack may have serious consequences for the future of occupational therapy.

It is suggested here that one reason for our failure, so far, clearly to establish a professional identity is that we have no widely accepted principles for our practice. We lack 'observed regularities of relationship' between occupational therapy intervention and the means of intervention; between the selection of these means and

149

the goals of intervention; or between these goals and the aspirations of our clients. Instead, we have been seduced into practice based on the reductionist medical model, wherein pathology and its relief become the aim of intervention, rather than the much broader aim of competence and the quality of life (e.g. see Shannon 1977).

Principles should not be confused with ethics. Professional ethics relate to the values held by a profession as a whole, and to the rules developed by that profession and used to judge the actions of practitioners in terms of 'right' and 'wrong' (see also Thompson 1990). Principles, on the other hand, offer summary statements about the practice of a profession. They pertain to regularities of relationship between one aspect of behaviour and another, which may be observed time after time, so that this relationship becomes accepted as a known characteristic of professional practice. It should then be possible for observers of our practice to say that occupational therapy practice *always* reflects this behaviour. Principled practice is not, thus, necessarily the same as ethical practice.

Principles for practice

The notion of principles for the practice of occupational therapy is not new. Dr William Dunton, one of the founders of occupational therapy in the United States, formulated the first such principles in 1918. Dunton's nine principles are listed in Box 6.1.

Box 6.1   Dunton's principles for practice

1. That work should be carried on with cure as the main object.
2. That work must be interesting.
3. The patient should be carefully studied.
4. That one form of occupation should not be carried out to the point of fatigue.
5. That it (the occupation) should have some useful end.
6. That it preferably should lead to an increase in the patient's knowledge.
7. That it should be carried out with other individuals.
8. That every possible encouragement should be given to the worker.
9. That work resulting in a poor or useless product is better than idleness.

Although Dunton's principles are presented as statements, or guidelines, it is possible to identify relationships between 'work' and 'cure' which reflect the notion that work is interesting, has a useful end, increases knowledge and mitigates against idleness. They also reflect relationships between the 'patient' and the 'therapist'. The patient is to be studied, protected from fatigue, encouraged, and preferably is to work in the company of others.

Writing some 60 years after Dunton, Reed & Sanderson (1980) proposed a further nine principles based on a conceptual model for practice-related personal adaptation through occupation (see Box 6.2).

Box 6.2   Reed et al's principles for practice

1. Occupational therapists can analyse with the client those occupations which will be most useful to the individual.
2. Occupational therapists can analyse the skills needed to perform specific occupations.
3. Occupational therapy can assess problems in skill development and acquisition by evaluating the functional components of motor, sensory, cognitive, intrapersonal and interpersonal performance.
4. Occupational therapy can predict problems in occupational performance based on the analysis of problems in skill development.
5. Occupational therapists can enable an individual to learn or re-learn skills required to perform the occupations which are needed by the individual.
6. Occupational therapy can assist the individual to integrate the skills needed to perform occupations.
7. Occupational therapy can enable an individual to adapt to the environment through the use of selected occupations.
8. Occupational therapy can assist the sociocultural environment to adapt to an individual through the use of selected occupations.
9. Occupational therapy can produce change in occupational performance and skill development faster than a person could obtain results using individual resources alone.

Three of Reed's suggested principles reflect the skills of the practitioner; the remaining six refer to the role of the profession. The practitioner is presented as skilled in the analysis of occupations deemed useful to the client, and in the analysis of those skills required to perform such occupations – in other words, skilled in both functional and task analysis. The practitioner is also presented as an enabler of learning. The profession is seen as focusing on assessment, the prediction of problems, the integration of skills, environmental and sociocultural adaptation, all in relation to 'occupation' with an expected outcome of enhancing the client's performance. In summary, Reed suggests principles identifying functional and task analysis by the practitioner as the means by which assessment, integration and adaptation may occur in order to enhance client performance.

The present authors, of course, support these ideas, but also suggest that principles for the practice of occupational therapy can be more clearly stated (Box 6.3).

Box 6.3   Proposed principles for practice

Principle 1   Occupational therapy intervention is through the use of activity.

Principle 2   The activity used in occupational therapy intervention is determined through functional analysis and task analysis.

Principle 3   The client is offered opportunities for learning so that a change in behaviour may occur.

Principle 4   The expected outcome of occupational therapy intervention reflects the goals of the client.

Of these four principles, the first relates to activity in its general sense as the profession's unique *means* of intervention. The second specifies the basis on which appropriate therapeutic activities are *selected*, while the third and fourth principles indicate that providing learning opportunities is the *method* by which occupational therapists endeavour to effect change, always taking into account the goals and aspirations of the client. These principles reflect that the practice of occupational therapy is based on the observation of a consistent or regular relationship between the goals of intervention and the means, selected means, and method of intervention; and that client goals are reflected in the overall goals of intervention (Fig. 6.1). They are thus a summary of the 'observed regularities' of our practice. By accepting them as such, observers of our practice would indeed be able to say that 'occupational therapy *always* intervenes by these means, using this method, and towards the aspirations of clients', and our professional identity would be clearly reflected and established. Box 6.4 looks more closely at these principles to help clarify reasons underlying what they propose (see also Fig. 6.2).

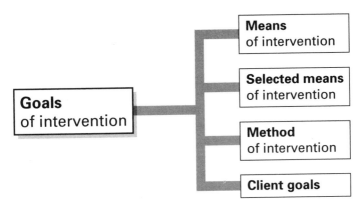

Fig. 6.1 Relationship between goals and intervention.

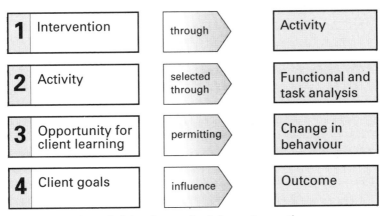

Fig. 6.2 The four principles of occupational therapy intervention.

Box 6.4   The four principles of practice: an expanded treatment

Principle 1   Occupational therapy intervention is through the use of activity.

We use activity as a means of intervention because:
- activity is the means, the measure and the outcome of normal growth and development
- health is determined by the functional activity of the individual (see Engelhardt 1974, Shannon 1977)
- engaging in activity changes the focus of attention from disability to the activity.

The concept of a change is crucial to understanding the unique role of occupational therapy. Other professions, such as physiotherapy, are extremely skilful in offering a programme of graded exercise which will improve elbow extension, fine-finger movement, or whatever. Many professions legitimately offer to teach relaxation, assertiveness skills or social skills. Occupational therapists are unique in that their intervention relies on literally 'diverting' the attention of clients from their present functional limitations to focus instead on an activity – a concrete task, which while requiring the same performance in terms of elbow extension, fine-finger movement, concentration, decision making or social interaction, also results in the production of a desired and desirable object whose making becomes the focus of attention. Everyone has experienced the phenomenon of a change in focus; has wanted, for example, to win a computer game or a set of tennis and has therefore ignored the physical aches and psychic stress inherent in the process. It is this concept of changing the focus, of diverting the attention from disability to the production of a concrete object, this observed regularity of relationship between occupational therapy and the use of activity which, it is suggested, forms a principle for the practice of occupational therapy.

Over the years, we, as a profession, have come to belittle 'diversional' occupational therapy, conferring on it a status far below that of those reductionist procedures which are more compatible with a medical model. This is a pity as we therefore throw away part of the uniqueness of our profession. A sound scientific base underlies the concept of changing focus, of diverting attention. All aspects of human motor development occur without our paying attention. Children run, hop and skip, engaging in activities which help to harden bone, develop muscle, integrate sensation. However, the child is paying attention to the activity requiring running, hopping or skipping, while the physiological processes take place without her knowledge. The same is true when change is the desired outcome of occupational therapy intervention. A correctly selected activity provides the focus of attention and the opportunity for learning, while the desired change can gradually occur. The client is not required, deliberately or consciously, to become more autonomous, or to extend the range of motion of an injured joint.

Principle 2   The activity used in occupational therapy intervention is determined through functional and task analysis.

The choice of a particular activity as occupational therapy depends on the current functional activity of the client, and on the requirements of the tasks needed to perform the activity. A knowledge of how these tasks may be graded, increased or decreased in their demands, and of how to match this grading to the changing functional ability of the client is a fundamental principle in the practice of occupational therapy. Functional and task analysis are discussed in detail in Chapter 8.

Principle 3   The client will be offered opportunities for learning so that a change in behaviour may occur.

In Chapter 3, it was suggested that one way for a change in behaviour to occur is through learning; that providing opportunities for learning is the nature of our practice. Learning an activity focuses the attention on the activity while, in order to perform the activity, learning also takes place at an unconscious level so that the therapeutic goal of remediation may occur. For example, in order to make a basket, the learning of such skills as randing, whaling, upsetting and keeping stakes parallel is required. In the language of the old basket makers' rhyme:

I can rand at your command
And set a tidy border.
I can upset tight
And whale alright
And keep my stakes in order.

The performance of these tasks requires hand-eye coordination, visual perception, complex fine-finger and wrist movements, concentration and judgement; all of these may be graded through the use of different weights of cane, as well as through size of the finished product and complexity of style. The outcome is *both* a useful finished product *and* enhancement of physical and intellectual performance.

Similarly, when engaging in a computer game, the participant needs to learn the skills of loading a cassette, manipulating switches in a particular sequence, and increasing speed. These activities require hand-eye coordination, finger and wrist dexterity, concentration and judgement, the requirements for which may be increased in order to grade the activity. The outcome is experiencing some measure of success, as well as the enhancement of performance. Computers may also, of course, be adapted for operation by head, mouth or feet, thus offering considerable flexibility.

In both of these examples, two types of learning take place: learning at the conscious level through focus on the activity, and learning at the sub-cortical or unconscious level, where the physical and/or intellectual performance will have been enhanced. The outcome of learning is not only change in specific aspects of behaviour. Learning an activity also permits, through the mastery of skills, a change in performance competence in physical, intellectual and psychosocial domains.

Principle 4   The expected outcome of occupational therapy intervention reflects the goals of the client.

Of the ten values of the profession proposed by Yerxa

(1980) – see Chapter 3 – eight reflect the perceptions we hold of our clients – their essential humanity, their self-directedness, their need to control their own environment, their potential and their participation in treatment. So far as the relationship between ourselves, as therapists, and our clients is concerned, a generalist (as opposed to a reductionist) view is adopted; we see the relationship as one of cooperation and, above all, recognise that our clients have every right to their own subjective perspective on the current reality of their condition. The goals of our clients must coincide with the expected outcome of our intervention, even when these goals appear to contradict our own preferences.

Gareth Williams (1984, 1986, 1987) reflects on both the medical and political issues impinging on the rehabilitation of the chronically disabled. His 1987 paper is specifically related to the assessment of activities of daily living, and is based on a previously published account of a study of individuals with rheumatoid arthritis. The issues he raises, however, are transferable to a wide range of clients. The paper makes the point that many ADL assessments comprise check lists premissed on the assumption that all the activities assessed carry equal weight. The items on such lists are seen out of context of the particular circumstances, or goals, of the individual being assessed. Williams states that this approach is 'empirical and inductive'. He further suggests that traditional approaches to assessment are 'limited in their utility because they abstract everyday activities from their context – and thereby empty them of their social significance'. The present authors concur with this view and also suggest that this type of reductionist assessment ignores the subjective goals of the individual, who may well be more interested in independence in one particular aspect of ADL than in others. For example, some clients prefer to be able to run a home-based business with the help of a computer and a telephone, and to use the money they so earn to buy services for cooking, cleaning and some aspects of personal care. It is the recognition of this subjective perspective of the client which becomes so vital, and which is reflected in the fourth principle of practice for occupational therapy. Sometimes, the client is not the same individual as the

designated patient. This is often the case with the elderly
or the chronically disabled when a relative is the primary
carer. It is the latter who then become our clients, and it
is their goals which we need to identify and help them
work towards achieving.

Conclusion

In conclusion, four principles have been proposed for the
practice of occupational therapy – four observed
regularities of relationship: between the means of practice
and the goals of practice; between the *selected* means of
practice and goals of practice; between the method of
practice and the goals of practice; and between the stated
goals of the client and the goals of practice. It was
recognised that to have stated principles for practice is not
a new idea, and we urged that these principles be accepted
and adhered to so that our practice may be identified,
recognised as unique and enhanced. The authors submit
that the principles suggested are compatible with the 'hard
core' of occupational therapy, that they are congruent with
the values, the authority, the knowledge, the nature and
the limits of practice (Ch. 3.) Further, it is suggested that
the theoretical frames of reference which protect the 'hard
core' adhere to these principles. All rely on activity as the
means of intervention, acknowledging that the precise
activity is selected through functional and task analysis;
they use learning as the method of intervention and they
accept the goals of the client as the goal of intervention.

7. Activity: its analysis and role in occupational therapy

INTRODUCTION

Occupation, activity, task, skill – all of these words are part of the vocabulary of occupational therapy and we tend to use them interchangeably. This is a pity, as each has its own meaning, distinct from that of the others. The issue of skills and their acquisition was addressed in Chapter 5. Occupation refers to that which occupies us between birth and death, and is sometimes, for convenience, classified into occupations relating to play, leisure, work and self-maintenance. Chambers' Dictionary (1983) defines 'activity' as 'the quality, state or fact of being active', and 'active' as 'in actual operation – in which the subject represents the doer of the action'. Tasks can be seen as segments of an activity, a sequence of tasks combining to form an activity.

Quite apart from occupational therapy's focus on activity, there can be little question that all forms of life are genetically programmed to be active on their own behalf. Plants absorb light and the chemicals they need for growth, and present themselves for pollination at the optimal time. Animals move around to meet their needs for food and shelter and to seek the best conditions for the rearing of their young. Humans are born with neurological reflexes sufficient to support life, and subsequently grow and develop through being active. Activity, then, is essential for the maintenance and continuance of life.

In Chapter 1, it was noted that various definitions of occupational therapy include the notion of activity. The American Occupational Therapy Association (AOTA) states that occupational therapy is 'the use of purposeful activity'. Turner (1981) states that occupational therapy is 'the treatment of the whole person through his active participation. . .'. More recently, the Committee of European Occupational Therapists (1989) suggested that 'purposeful activity' is the means through which clients are assessed and treated. Chapter 3 discussed the values of occupational therapy as relating to the client 'acting on his environment', and being 'productive'. In that same chapter it was suggested that part of our knowledge stems from an understanding of activity and the part this plays as the means, the measure and the outcome of normal growth and development. One of the principles of occupational therapy stated in Chapter 6 was that 'occupational therapy intervention is through the use of activity'.

The significance of activity in the proper practice of occupational therapy is thus clearly recognised in our public statements about ourselves, as a principle of our practice, as a part of our values, and as a contribution to the knowledge from which practice derives. Activity and the analysis of activity is a focal issue for occupational therapists. Much has been written on the subject and some remarkable claims have been made. In 1979, AOTA passed a resolution stating that 'purposeful activity includes both an intrinsic and a therapeutic purpose'. Llorens (1981) suggests that the intrinsic purpose of activity is derived from the response elicited by the activity and experienced by the performer of the activity in terms of affect, cognition and sensorimotor performance. Mosey (1981) sees activity analysis as an essential tool of occupational therapy, and considers that this analysis seeks to determine the distinctive characteristics of activities as well as their potential impact on individuals. Other writers, including Clark (1979) and Cynkin (1990) suggest that activity analysis is derived from a theory suggesting that activities have inherent characteristics, and that it is these characteristics which elicit specific responses from individuals engaged in them. However, as has also been observed in the literature, Stein (1979) notes that 'this inherent quality of activity has received little attention' (from the profession of occupational therapy).

One attempt to test these ideas was reported by Boyer et al (1989). Their study sought to test the hypothesis that activities have inherent characteristics that can elicit similar affective responses. They identified four activities as the focus of their study: working with clay, leather lacing, filing and using an 'exercycle'. Their conclusions provide statistical support for some of the commonsense, clinically derived theories of occupational therapy, documenting a difference between the affective response to a highly structured activity (filing) and that to an unstructured, non-directed activity (working with clay). They suggest that further research is needed to refine our understanding of the specific elements of activities which most influence the affective responses of individuals.

Until such time as this refinement may occur, the present authors would suggest a less complex and more pragmatic view of activity analysis which comprises two distinct parts: (1) an analysis of the activity itself; and (2) an analysis of the current functional ability of the individual performing the activity. It is suggested that some of what has previously been written on the subject of activity analysis has tended to confuse these separate issues and has, as a consequence, attempted to assign to an activity, attributes more properly assigned to the doer of the activity.

ANALYSIS OF ACTIVITY

Activity does not require consciousness and is not specific to humans. In many instances it may be performed by a robot. An activity comprises a sequence of tasks, which are the requirements of the activity. These tasks and the sequence in which they occur do not vary. They remain the same regardless of who (or what) performs them. For example, the sequence of tasks in the activity of pouring tea from a pot is:

- the handle of the pot must be grasped.
- the pot must be lifted.
- the pot must be tilted.

There can be no question that any human agent performing this activity requires sufficient sensorimotor ability to grasp, to lift and to tilt. The task also requires cognitive ability for learning and/ or performance. However, to suggest that the activity of pouring tea from a pot will elicit affective responses which (a) can be measured, or (b) will be transferable from one individual to another or, indeed, are likely to be the same for any individual from one occasion to another is clearly nonsense. Affective response to an activity depends on the age, past experience and current mood of the individual concerned, as well as on the influence of the society and culture within which the activity is taking place. All these factors may be as diverse as the individual performers themselves.

Activity may be analysed in terms of:
1. permanent and unchanging requirements intrinsic to the activity itself

2. other requirements, such as those of space, equipment and materials, which are always present and need consideration, but which change
3. social and cultural perceptions of both the activity and the outcome of the activity.

1. Requirements intrinsic to the activity itself include:

- a list of tasks in their most logical sequence
- the sensorimotor requirements of each task
- the cognitive requirements of each task.

2. Other permanent requirements of the activity are those involving:

- space. An activity requires space for its performance; the space required depends on such changing factors as the size of the operator, whether the operator stands, sits, uses crutches or is wheelchair-bound. Space also relates to the equipment to be used: for example, the space required to clean a window depends, in part, on the size of the window and whether or not a ladder is to be used.
- equipment. Most activities require equipment. This depends not only on the activity, but also on the operator's current functional abilities (see section on 'Grading and adaptation' below).
- materials. All activities in occupational therapy require the use of materials, but here again the exact type and amount of materials needed varies, depending both on the desired outcome of the activity and on what is available. Locally produced materials are often the most appropriate. This is particularly true for cooking activities.
- cost of materials and equipment. This needs to be known and clearly depends on the appropriate equipment and materials.

3. Concerning social and cultural perceptions of the performance of an activity, Cynkin (1990) offers a sociocultural classification of activities which includes learning from generation to generation, emphasis on the family as a socialising influence, and the value which societies place on tradition and ritual. This classification is useful, although it is suggested that attention should be given to the social perception of the performance of a given activity and also of its outcome. For example, in some sociocultural strata, window cleaning is perceived as 'man's work' or work that is paid for, while

having clean windows is regarded as essential. In other strata of the same culture, the actual cleaning of windows may be perceived as an honourable aspect of good housekeeping. In other cultures, the entire concept of window cleaning is non-existent – for example, igloos or the native dwellings of tropical societies do not have windows. An understanding of the cultural norms and of the varying socio-economic perceptions of activities are important factors in the analysis of activity (Fig. 7.1).

An example of the application of the above suggestions to the analysis of an activity – that of stool seating – is given in Box 7.1 and Figure 7.2.

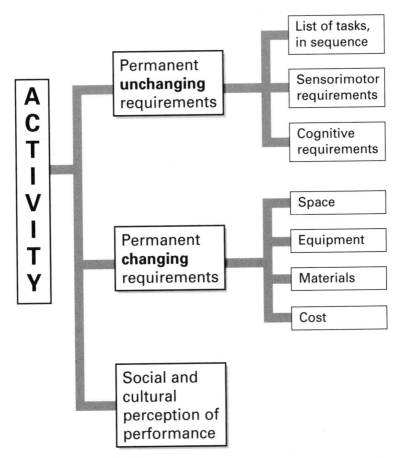

Fig. 7.1 Analysis of activity.

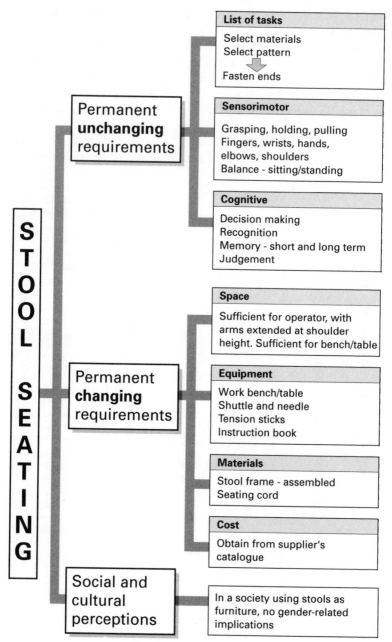

Fig. 7.2 Stool seating: activity analysis.

Box 7.1   Analysing the activity of stool seating

1. The permanent, unchanging requirements intrinsic to the activity include the following:

● *List of tasks in their most logical sequence:*
   - select materials, e.g. colour of seating cord
   - select pattern to be woven
   - secure end of cord to lower rung of stool
   - place tension sticks
   - commence winding cord around upper rung of stool and across top of stool in sequence required for chosen pattern
   - secure final end of cord to lower rung of stool
   - remove tension sticks
   - turn stool
   - secure end of cord to lower rung of stool
   - load cord onto shuttle, or thread through eye of seating needle
   - weave cord through strands already in place in format required by chosen pattern
   - secure final end of cord to lower rung of stool
   - thread all four ends of cord through underside of strands
   - fasten ends to secure.

● *The sensorimotor requirements of each task:*
   - grasping, holding, pulling
   - fingers, wrist, hands, elbow, shoulder
   - balance – either sitting or standing.

● *The cognitive requirements of tasks:*
   - decision making
   - recognition
   - memory – short-term and long-term
   - judgement.

2. Other requirements:
● *Space.* Should be sufficient for operator, either seated or standing, with arms extended at shoulder height. Sufficient space also required for work bench or table.

- *Equipment*
  - work bench or table
  - shuttle and seating cord needle
  - tension sticks
  - instruction book, giving choice of pattern.
- *Materials*
  - stool frame – assembled
  - seating cord.
- *Cost.* Obtain from supplier's catalogue.

3. Social and cultural perceptions of the activity and its outcome. In any society which has a use for a stool as an article of furniture, the activity of seating a stool carries no gender-related implications. It is an androgynous activity.

ANALYSIS OF THE CURRENT FUNCTIONAL ABILITY OF THE INDIVIDUAL PERFORMING AN ACTIVITY

An ever-increasing library of assessment tools for occupational therapy is being developed and published. Some of these are standardised, some are of the 'check list' variety, some fall within a particular frame of reference, some require interpretation by the therapist, some are recommended for specific forms of dysfunction (e.g. physical, psychiatric, mental handicap), or for the happier functioning of the elderly. All are welcomed, although it is no part of the focus of this book to review or evaluate them; most are included in professional publications and are readily available. All certainly have their uses, although many focus on pathology which, in many instances, has been identified as such by one or more members of a health care profession. Many ignore the sociocultural framework within which the client lives, and most disregard the subjective perspective of the client.

This being the case, there would seem to be some value in starting the process of functional analysis by asking the client how he normally spends his waking life. This idea was suggested in 1965 by Richard Spahr and is included in Hemphill's (1982) book on evaluation in psychiatric occupational therapy. The present authors have, over the years, found this strategy invaluable in helping clients to identify the activities in which they engage, hour by hour, day by day, for a typical week of their normal lives. Having completed this first stage, they are asked to rate each activity on a scale from 'most essential' to 'least necessary', and then again on a scale from 'most enjoyed' to 'most disliked'. Finally, the client and therapist together have some data to work with and may identify what, in the client's view, needs to be changed. This will, of course, vary: it may be the restoration of needed function currently lost through trauma; the finding of alternative methods for necessary function where no restoration is likely (both of which require precise assessment); the assessment of cognitive abilities such as concentration, memory or judgement; the assessment of interactive ability; or whatever else the client and therapist together identify as the deficit in the client's functional needs the correction of which would improve his ability to pursue his own life. It then becomes the therapist's role to 'give advice and to be heard' as she identifies the most appropriate frame of reference within which the client may seek change through learning, and, as a first step in this process, administers the best assessment instrument available.

THE ROLE OF ACTIVITY

The role of activity in the intervention offered by occupational therapy is, we suggest, allied to the usual procedures followed in the majority of occupational therapy services.

Reed's (1980) outline of the procedures followed in occupational therapy is given in Box 7.2.

Box 7.2   Reed's outline of procedures

1. *Referral of client to occupational therapy.* Comes from a variety of sources.
2. *Initial screening.* The purpose of this screening is, of course, to identify the client's needs, and decide whether or not occupational therapy intervention is likely to help meet those needs. The method used for initial screening could well follow that suggested by Spahr (see above), whereby the client shares the activities pursued in his or her everyday life, thus making possible the

3. *Assessment of need*. Clients' self-identified needs are highlighted, leading to

4. *Acceptance of client (or not) for occupational therapy.*

5. *Specific evaluation of identified needs.* This may be implemented through existing tests or through the use of activities. In and of themselves, most activities are excellent specific evaluation tools. For example, grasp may be evaluated through the handling of equipment and materials, such as plants, seedlings, needles and shuttles, pencils, paint brushes or woodwork tools. Strength may be evaluated through the use of block-printing, various gardening procedures and woodwork. Short-term memory may be evaluated by teaching the client a simple procedure which is new to him, and concentration by asking the client to complete a simple set of procedures within a given time.

   In many instances, the use of activity is the most satisfactory way of conducting a specific evaluation of the client's present functional ability. This kind of evaluation may be tailor-made and, where it seems appropriate, designed to incorporate such variables as working alone, in a small group or as a member of a larger one. The observational skills of the therapist are legitimately exercised, and opportunities arise for non-verbal clues offered by the client to be pursued. This is not always the case when a more scientifically structured form of evaluation is used.

6. *Programme planning* is a combined undertaking of the client and the therapist. Needs have been identified and a plan is now made: a plan which is interesting, stimulating and even exciting for the client, within a frame of reference, and focusing on attaining desired change in specific function through some form of learning. The disabled housewife should not be expected to spend her time in occupational therapy practising cooking or cleaning. What could be more boring or more disheartening than to struggle along, inadequately performing household tasks which had formerly been accomplished easily, skilfully and

quickly? Filling, lifting and carrying containers of water can just as well be relearned with jars for painting as with saucepans for vegetables. The client may not only regain needed everyday skills but also, perhaps, enlarge her repertoire of leisure and pleasurable activities.

7. *Intervention* is the implementation of the plans formulated by client and therapist.
8. *Reassessment* is necessary at frequent intervals, partly to measure the change which has occurred in the client's functional ability, and partly to offer an occasion for
9. *Possible modification of the original plan and the chosen intervention strategies*. Reassessment is most wisely conducted using the same tool as was used for the original specific screening; decisions may then be made regarding the grading of activity already being used or the introduction of a different activity.
10. *Discharge of the client* from occupational therapy.

GRADING AND ADAPTATION

The concepts of grading and adaptation are important within the practice of occupational therapy. Grading is of interest in the planning and implementation phases, and following reassessment. Activities may be graded so that their demands increase as functional ability increases. Grading may be in terms of complexity, size, time allowed for completion and speed of completion of the activity. For example, the activity of gardening may be graded from the planting of seedlings in a prepared container, through the preparation of a container, to digging and preparing a garden bed. This grading of activity requires the increase of a number of functional abilities, including grasp, strength, concentration and memory. The flexibility inherent in the possibilities for grading activities is one of the assets of using activities as the means of occupational therapy practice.

Just as grading refers to activity, so adaptation refers to equipment and architectural structures. Equipment may be adapted in order to change its size and/or shape. For example, cutlery may be adapted, as may the handles of tools. The height of working surfaces or of seating arrangements may be adapted to suit the particular requirements of individual clients. Again, it is the flexibility permitted by adaptation which enhances the possibilities inherent in occupational therapy intervention. The removal or modification of structural barriers in private dwellings or in public institutions is adaptation on a somewhat grander scale. The purpose of adaptation is that clients may better pursue the activities they choose as part of their normal lives.

In summary, activity plays a pre-eminent role in the assessment, the planning and the implementation of occupational therapy. The purpose of occupational therapy is that clients may be active in their own lives and helped to develop, to increase or to enhance their own health.

8. Work and leisure

The concept of activity embraces work and leisure pursuits and the self-care skills of daily living. The term's broad scope acknowledges that work, leisure and self-maintenance have much in common. Each of these areas of life satisfies fundamental human needs, and each involves activities that contribute to feelings of self-worth, independence and competence. Today, the common ground shared by work and leisure is easily overlooked, and they are often seen as polar opposites. The implication is that while work is constructive, leisure is not, an assumption which is invalid. For all of us, experience of leisure, in the form of childhood play, predates that of work. Far from being passive, play contributes constructively to many aspects of development.

PLAY

In play, children engage in activities that offer fun and enjoyment. Although play is rewarding in its own right, it nevertheless serves several useful functions: it enhances curiosity, imagination and cognitive development generally; it provides a forum for practising social roles and skills; and it offers an outlet for physical energy and pent-up emotions. Piaget observed that play begins early in the sensorimotor period, when the infant repeats actions that are pleasurable. Imitative play emerges with the onset of primitive representations. At first, the child enjoys copying the actions of people in his immediate environment but, at roughly 18 months, deferred imitation also becomes possible. Finally, towards the end of the second year, pretend play appears in the repertoire. Initially, everyday objects are used symbolically – as when the child uses a block to represent a car, while moving it along the ground and saying 'beep-beep'. Simple substitutive play of this kind paves the way for more advanced forms of make-believe. The pretend play of pre-school children centres on role-taking. They may play at being parents, teachers or pop stars, thus acting out their feelings about authority and discipline, and learning more about adult roles in the process.

Parten (1972) identified several categories of play (Fig. 8.1). Less social forms include:

- *unoccupied* – random, no clear goal. Child may stand in one place or walk around the room
- *solitary* – child concentrates on what she is doing but plays alone and pays no attention to other children
- *onlooker* – child watches other children's play with interest and may engage in conversation but does not take part
- *parallel* – child plays with the same toys as other children and may imitate their play but nevertheless child actually plays alone

while two further types – *associative* and *cooperative* play – are grounded in social interaction. As development proceeds, solitary activities decrease, and play becomes more socially oriented. The associative play of pre-school children is based on common group activity, but it remains poorly organised and there is little agreement on goals and rules. Only towards the end of the pre-operational period does play become truly cooperative and rooted

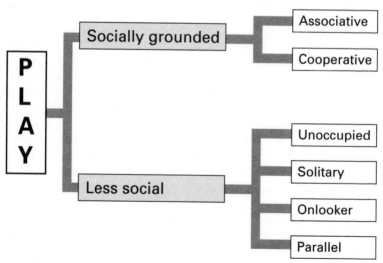

Fig. 8.1 Parten's categories of play.

in a sense of group identity. Now goals and roles are worked out by consensus, and games are organised according to agreed rules of procedure.

There is a good deal of evidence in favour of Piaget's claim that play is adaptive. Connolly (1982) has found that pre-school children who favour pretend play perform better than do controls in Piagetian tests of cognitive development; it has also been found that toddlers who frequently engage in exploratory play have an advantage five years later over their peers in tests of creativity, independence and curiosity (Hutt & Bhavani, 1976). Independence and curiosity are known to characterise creative adults, as do the traits of flexibility and cognitive complexity (Barron 1969, Quinn 1980). Thus, it may be that there is some kind of connection between play experiences in childhood and creativity in later life. Anne Roe's classical study of eminent American scientists (1952) found that most reported loneliness and isolation in their early years – a circumstance which implies greater than average opportunities to play with and explore 'things' as opposed to people. In her later writings on vocational development, Roe suggests that childhood experiences of this kind will influence the direction and field of adult achievement. However, her views, although interesting, remain speculative as they are based on retrospective accounts which may be unreliable.

Rubin et al (1983) have reviewed numerous studies of play and its correlates, and have concluded that play does indeed help to foster social and cognitive skills. Theorists concerned with education also acknowledge the constructive nature of play. Piaget's claim (1951) that children are active in their own learning has encouraged teachers to abandon traditional rote-learning procedures in favour of discovery-learning techniques which challenge the child's interest and curiosity. Likewise, the philosophies of Froebel and Montessori have focused on play and the use of concrete, age-appropriate materials as means of exploiting the child's natural desire for knowledge.

Work and its rewards

Conceptualisations of work change radically from age to age, and generally reflect the economic and social circumstances of a particular era. In Ancient Greece, manual work was considered demeaning. The Greeks thought of philosophy and rhetoric as noble pursuits and work as the business of slaves. The idea that

Box 8.1   Reilly's Studies of Play

Play is a universal phenomenon. It is not confined to childhood; 'playfulness' remains with us throughout life. To be deprived of playful experiences retards competent function – but why? What is play, and why does playful behaviour generate the tools of mastery? In 'Play as exploratory learning' (1974) Mary Reilly notes that the very obviousness of play has precluded serious scientific inquiry as to what it is. She suggests that any explanation of play must include knowledge based in biology, psychology, sociology and anthropology, so that a multidimensional approach is required.

Play and learning

Reilly proposes a general systems theory approach in which play is seen as essentially part of the learning process – in fact the means through which the building blocks of learning are acquired. Early 'hapinstantial' play forms the initial schemata which are gradually added to and expanded to provide a structure for all subsequent learning. The sensorimotor play engaged in by infants exploring themselves and their environment, which asks the question 'what is this?', establishes the very first learning experience. Gradually, the infant becomes able to adapt to objects in the environment; adaptation occurs to the process of feeding, to tactile experience and to his own and other people's motor responses. This learning increases as the child begins to receive and give communication through sound, and eventually language, and play is used for practice, through repetition, towards mastery. Mastery of any kind requires the learning of rules which govern skill, and Reilly suggests that play is again the means through which the child discovers, tests and learns these rules. The capacity for imaginative or pretend play is yet another way of learning, of answering the question, 'what would happen if?'

Play deprivation

To be deprived of play experiences, because of either

physical limitations or environmental deficiencies, can seriously inhibit learning opportunities, with resulting poverty in the initial schemata of infancy. Although studies have been reported, by Reilly's students among others, identifying the limitations evident in individuals deprived of play experiences, there are as yet few studies setting norms in mastery skills among those who are not thus deprived. Nonetheless, the inclusion of play and of activities based on playful behaviour have always been part of the tradition of occupational therapy practice.

work could be intrinsically satisfying gained ground in the Middle Ages with the rise of the artisan class. Craftsmen enjoyed a high degree of autonomy, and took pride in creating a finished product. This attitude changed in the wake of the industrial revolution. Creative participation in work declined with mechanisation, and Marxist philosophy highlighted people's alienation from the product of their labour. Technological developments in today's post-industrial world have made many skills redundant. The resulting scarcity of jobs has created a climate in which work is possibly overevaluated. The high value placed on work, relative to leisure, is underpinned by the residual influence of the Protestant work ethic.

Early research

Research into the rewards of work began in earnest during the first half of this century. At the outset, interest in the area largely reflected the problems posed to management by rapid organisational growth and the need to motivate an expanding work-force. Early research was based on the assumption that people had little natural inclination to work. It was believed that disciplinary measures and productivity-based payment schemes were the best inducements, although many firms did make efforts to improve physical conditions in the work-place. Within the incentive tradition, Frederick ('Speedy') Taylor (1947) showed that specially selected workers could be induced to quadruple their output when paid to carry out instructions to the letter. His studies – forerunners to modern time-and-motion techniques – placed all responsibility for task design with management, allowing none to the employee.

Box 8.2 The Mayo experiment

The classic experiment to challenge the view that physical conditions were all-important was carried out in the late 1920s by Elton Mayo at the Hawthorne Plant near Chicago. Mayo found that productivity did increase with changes in working conditions (better illumination, rest pauses, shorter working hours and so on) but continued to rise even when these were reversed. Clearly, the girls who participated in the study felt differently about their work once they were consulted and their cooperation sought, and it was this factor that lay behind the rise in output.

Herzberg: hygienes and motivators

Herzberg (1974) has made a useful distinction between the factors that contribute to job satisfaction and those that contribute to dissatisfaction. His view, based on his own research, is that satisfaction and dissatisfaction at work are separate dimensions, and not two ends of a single continuum. Some factors, which he names *'hygienes'* 'serve primarily to prevent job dissatisfaction, while having little effect on positive job attitudes'. Such factors include *company policy, supervision, interpersonal relations* and *working conditions*. When these are low, employees are discontented, but improvements in these areas are valuable only to a point. Concentrating attention on hygiene factors fails to provide for positive satisfaction because 'they do not possess the characteristics necessary for giving the individual a sense of growth' (Herzberg 1974). Factors that do relate to reports of high job satisfaction are termed 'motivators', and include such determinants as *achievement, recognition, responsibility* and *the nature of work* itself.

Herzberg's theory has inspired a great deal of research, not all of which is favourable to his thesis. Studies which have failed to replicate his results, however, are generally those that take a traditional unidimensional view of job satisfaction, and do not use the recommended investigatory procedures. Thus, disputes about the two-factor theory too often focus on the issue of methodology, which is hardly relevant to the present theme. More important is the fact that researchers employing the appropriate methodology have at times found that, for some groups, factors originally identified as hygienes may, in fact, contribute to positive job attitudes (Gardner 1977). In his 1974 review of replications to date, Herzberg acknowledges this, and draws attention to two such studies – one using industrial supervisors, the other professional women employed in government – in which interpersonal relationships at work were found to function as motivators, not merely as factors preventing discontent. However, in other respects, these, and a host of other replications, have tended to corroborate Herzberg's main predictions. In an early review of 16 critical investigations, Whitsett & Winslow (1967) observed that many studies purporting to be critical yielded results that actually support the theory, at least in part, and they concluded that Herzberg's theory retains its utility and viability. There is, then, a great deal of evidence to substantiate Herzberg's claim that the factors which genuinely motivate people at work are those that relate to a positive self-concept and the individual's sense of growth.

Work and the self concept

Throughout the individual's working life, a reciprocal relationship exists between work and the self-concept. Even in early adolescence, the young person's sense of identity influences career aspirations.

Super

In a number of influential publications, Donald Super has contended that finding a career is never a matter of making simple choices. He argues in favour of a vocational development perspective, in which adjustment is a more relevant concept than choice. The origins of vocational adjustment are, he claims, rooted in childhood, when occupational roles are acted out in fantasy and play. During adolescence, aspirations become more realistic, and the individual more aware that compromise may be required. Role-playing – in leisure occupations, part-time work, counselling interviews and other activities – helps to develop interests and preferences; and it continues to influence adjustment even when the person is established in the world of work. Super is strongly committed to the view that vocational development is a life-long process: we develop even as we choose to leave our jobs, accept promotion or make decisions about retirement. He has identified five life-stages: *growth, exploration, establishment, maintenance* and *decline*. Exploration is of most interest to career counsellors, because it coincides with adolescence. This stage embodies *fantasy* and *tentative* subphases, and concludes with the *crystallisation* of attitudes that accompanies increased realism and self-knowledge.

Super's theory is, above all, an elaboration of the proposition that the process of vocational development is essentially that of *developing and implementing a self-concept* (Super 1965). Over a life-time, the individual plays roles in leisure and work through which he tests out his abilities and compares his own achievements and preferences with those of others. Gradually, these reflections of self grow into a more consistent self-concept which the person seeks to preserve and enhance through a number of activities, especially those in the occupational field. The choice of an occupation is one of the points in life at which a young person is required to state in fairly explicit terms his concept of self. Thereafter, satisfaction relates to whether an occupation remains compatible with the developing self-concept and permits the individual to play the kind of role he finds congenial and appropriate.

Alternative views

While self-concept and occupational development are clearly intertwined, the question arises whether this aspect of self does, in fact, play the determining role Super assigns to it. For example, Warnath (1979) is extremely critical of the idea that the individual with adequate motivation, information and guidance can move through the educational process and find job goals that allow for implementation of the self-concept. He objects to theories that emphasise fulfilment and self-actualisation, since only a minority of jobs are capable of engaging one's fully human qualities. These theories, moreover, have little regard for factors of race and social status that limit choice, and they overlook environmental constraints, such as unemployment and the realities of the economic system.

A great many firms have, in fact, tried to redesign work in ways that satisfy higher level needs. Job-enrichment programmes have increased in the western world, as have efforts to enhance employee responsibility, Nevertheless, it remains the case that jobs of higher socio-economic status are far more likely to offer personal fulfilment. Havinghurst (1982) found that less skilled workers in low status jobs identified payment as the factor that gave most meaning to their work, whereas more privileged groups did not. Likewise, according to the 1973 Upjohn Institute survey, American professional and white-collar workers were twice as likely as blue-collar workers to state that, given the chance, they would choose the same type of work again.

Work and rehabilitation

Although only a small proportion of people taking part in an occupational therapy programme will be able to return to paid employment, teaching work-related activities remains an important part of the therapist's repertoire. In order to help clients with good prospects for open or sheltered employment, the therapist must relate presenting performance deficits to previous experience. Making this kind of connection may involve taking account of the person's cultural background and values, in addition to assessing work-related abilities. Hobbs Cubie et al (1985) have pointed out that spinal cord injury patients whose backgrounds place a high value on sport and physical achievement will need a different programme emphasis from similarly injured patients whose cultures value intellectual achievement. Likewise, hand injuries may have different consequences for blue-and white-collar workers. For the former, injury is likely to involve loss of the work role; the latter group may only have to make some adjustments.

Nichol

Nichol (1984) writing in the context of short-term psychiatric care, suggests that when they are appropriate, work-related activities should be introduced progressively to help build up 'concentration, memory, manual dexterity, initiative, stamina and interpersonal relationships, all of which are usually required to function in a job'. Alternatively, depending on the circumstances, placement in a work unit might be advisable. Here the client can engage in clerical, industrial or manual work, as appropriate. The occupational therapist encourages desirable work habits and must liaise with team members and staff in other units to report on progress and discuss any further training, assessment and placement requirements that may arise. Nichol acknowledges, however, that in the absence of full employment many patients, regardless of their expressed desire to work, will never do so again. For this reason, she advises occupational therapists to be cautious when planning work-oriented programmes, for fear of instilling expectations that cannot realistically be fulfilled.

Kielhofner

Kielhofner (1985) defines occupation in broad terms as 'the output of the open system', and notes that work is but one of three forms of occupation, the other two being daily-living tasks and play. Each form of occupation may be carried out in healthy or unhealthy ways. Current conceptualisations of health, he points out, emphasise engagement in activity commensurate with capacity, the ability to meet environmental challenges and participation in work and play. Function, in this view, is more important than structure. Occupational therapists should therefore concern themselves with 'the adaptation of persons in terms of their occupational function and dysfunction' (p 63). He proposes a function/dysfunction continuum to guide assessment of a person's performance. Levels of occupational function include *achievement, competence* and *exploration,* while the three levels of dysfunction relate to *inefficacy, incompetence* and *helplessness.* Each of these levels can be evaluated in terms of the concepts that form the core of his model of human occupation (i.e. in terms of personal causation, interests, values, roles, habits, skills and the open system cycle). These, and a number of additional concepts, can also be used to analyse the nature and value of occupations.

Hobbs Cubie

Sally Hobbs Cubie (1985) has used Kielhofner's model to analyse meal preparation in terms of environment, volition, habituation, performance and output – thus providing an example of an activity that does not easily fit a work/non-work dichotomy. Her output analysis points to three aspects of the activity: work, play and daily living. Meal preparation obviously relates to self-maintenance and can relate to paid employment – for example, that of chefs and caterers. It also relates to play, in that parties frequently centre on food, and cooking is a hobby for many people. Hobbs Cubie writes that adaptive occupational behaviour requires a balance between work, play and daily-living tasks. She suggests that balance in the three areas of output should be reflected in treatment programmes.

Shepherd

The convention of defining work in purely economic terms means that many fairly laborious forms of activity are not looked upon as 'real' work if they are unpaid. (Hence the question, 'Do you work or are you a housewife?') Bearing in mind the distinction between employment as an economic relationship and work as a structured activity, Shepherd (1981) has written a thought-provoking paper on psychological disorder and lack of employment. He points out that individuals with established psychological disorder are most vulnerable to the effects of unemployment 'or at least the lack of structured activity', and notes that for this group 'being unemployed and being out of work amount to much the same thing' (p 345). Even when treatment is received, psychological symptoms are more likely to persist in the absence of work. Shepherd draws attention to studies in Britain by Brown and his coworkers on this issue. These have indicated that inactivity exacerbates the problems of chronic psychotic patients (Wing & Brown 1970) and that whole- or part-time work has protective value for women affected by depression (Brown & Harris 1978). Following the 1944 Disabled Person's Act, a number of provisions were made for resettlement. These included Employment Rehabilitation Centres, sheltered factories and the employment of several hundred Disablement Resettlement Officers. Wansbrough & Cooper (1980) reviewed their effectiveness with respect to people with mental illness, and their conclusions indicated how little the health authorities and social services actually contributed.

Wansbrough & Cooper included the failure of the quota system in their critique. Theoretically, medium-to-large firms should include 3% registered disabled persons among their employees. However, this was found to be rare, and Area Health Authorities to be as remiss as other bodies. In 1977, two-thirds of these authorities employed less than 1% disabled persons in their work force, the remaining one-third employing less than 2%. As far as the Employment Resettlement Centres were concerned, these catered primarily for the physically disabled. Generally they offered a maximum of one-quarter of their places to people with psychiatric problems. Re-employ factories offered sheltered work to thousands of disabled people but, again, only about 20% of these had psychiatric disability.

It is as yet too early to say whether the Disabled Persons (Services, Consultation and Rehabilitation) Act 1986 will be more effective and wide-ranging in application. It specifies rights to representation, consultation and advocacy, and offers disabled people a legal framework for equal participation in society. To date, the Act is by no means fully implemented and its focus remains on personal social services. However, when fully implemented, it will at least give people the right to have a say in decisions affecting their lives, whether these relate to employment opportunities or provisions of a more general nature.

Shepherd (1981) acknowledges that opportunities for open employment are likely to remain limited for those with a psychiatric condition, and he suggests that day-care centres are the most suitable places in which to provide appropriate occupations. He emphasises the therapeutic value of work-oriented activities on several grounds: they structure time, distract people from their problems, and offer social contact, friendship and other social rewards. Work also relates to self-esteem and a feeling of 'normality'. It may, in addition, provide money and job satisfaction. He contends that, although leisure activities can provide some of these rewards, they are generally less effective, especially in fostering social involvement. He quotes a study by Miles (1972) which examined improvements in social interaction among long-stay patients. It was found that the industrial unit was more effective in promoting improvement than was 'traditional occupational therapy'.

UNEMPLOYMENT

Research in the area of unemployment has strengthened two assumptions: (1) that work is equivalent to paid employment; and (2) that, given the undesirable effects of unemployment, paid work is essential for healthy psychological adjustment. We have already rejected the notion that work, to be perceived as work, must involve payment. Such a view involves excluding housework, child care, voluntary work, care of the elderly, gardening and so forth from the arena of work – an exclusion which is patently unacceptable. The assumption that unemployment necessarily brings psychological ill-effects in its wake is also open to question. Although unemployment is disastrous for many, one cannot be sure that it always has adverse psychological consequences. Often, psychological disturbance causes, or at least contributes to, the loss of a job and makes it more difficult for the person to find new work after a period of enforced inactivity. Given that studies of unemployment are non-experimental in design, all that they can establish is that some sort of relationship exists between unemployment and psychological upset. They cannot of their nature say that disturbance causes unemployment, nor that it is a consequence of the situation.

Gurney & Taylor (1981) have noted that current perspectives on unemployment are highly influenced by work carried out in the wake of the 1930s' Depression. They assert that this type of work has little relevance to today's situation. Firstly, research in the 1930s was flawed: sampling procedures left a lot to be desired, and control groups were not used. Secondly, loss of work today has less catastrophic consequences than during the Great Depression. Gurney & Taylor state that, in view of the cause-and-effect dilemma, many studies have failed to isolate a definite set of psychological effects that 'inevitably and universally accompanies unemployment'. Despite this failure, the belief persists that the psychological impact of unemployment is fully understood, as does the belief that 'such devastating consequences as plummetting self-esteem, rising drug addiction, alienation, despair and suicide are inevitable for all who become unemployed' (Gurney & Taylor 1981, p 350). These authors acknowledge that their objective view of the evidence may appear callous, but they argue that uncritical acceptance of 'received opinion' may lead to self-fulfilling prophecies on the part of the employed and unemployed alike. As things stand, the unemployed are too often viewed as a homogenous group, whereas studies of specific sub-groups have found that some such groups adapt to their circumstances with little or no apparent difficulty (e.g. Little 1976, Hartley 1980).

Since studies of unemployment cannot show conclusively that unemployment inevitably brings about psychological ill-effects, it cannot be concluded from these that paid work is essential for psychological well-being. Earlier in this chapter, it was seen that only certain types of work are truly motivating in that they offer rewards consistent with self-fulfilment. People stay in less satisfying jobs simply because they offer financial compensation and other 'hygiene' types of incentive. Increasingly, people in repetitive, unchallenging jobs seek personal fulfilment in leisure occupations. Even Shepherd – an ardent advocate of work-related activities – acknowledges that if people were paid to 'engage in leisure activities, then this would be progress indeed' (Shepherd 1981, p 347). Nichol (1984), along with many health care professionals, advocates a balance in life and in therapy between work, leisure pursuits and the activities of daily living. Moreover, the expressed needs of disabled persons often focus on leisure activities over and above those that relate to work. For example, assessment of the needs of Irish Wheelchair Association members (Faughnan 1977) found that 58.3% of the sample surveyed identified social contact and holidays as their most urgent need. The second most urgent need was for the provision of aids to assist independence (15.5%). The need for training geared to sheltered or home industry employment ranked third on the list, 12.1% of subjects expressing this as their most urgent requirement. 6.4% of subjects expressed significant interest in sport, travel and youth activities. In view of findings such as this, leisure activities clearly play an important role in rehabilitation.

LEISURE

Technological advances and economic circumstances have combined in the modern world to offer more people more leisure than at any other time in recent history. Although there have always been privileged classes who enjoyed more leisure than the rest of the population, modern society is characterised by wide access to this area of life. Reasons offered for this trend generally point to the fact that, as improved technology has reduced the amount of labour required to produce goods and services and production has become more efficient and profitable, so people have more free time and energy due to the shorter working week, and more money available for spending. Of course, this trend is not wholly beneficial. The more efficient the means of production, the fewer the numbers of people required for the work-force. Redundancies, early retirement and unemployment abound in our post-industrial society, so that, for many people, extra free time is enforced. Whether this increase is valued or judged to be an unwelcome consequence of illness or unemployment, there remains the problem of how best to adapt. The question of whether it is possible to enjoy one's free time without feeling guilty also arises in view of the pervasiveness of the work ethic.

Leisure can include any number of activities, including children's play, sport, even attending evening classes if attendance is pleasing and a matter of choice. There is no clear dividing line between leisure occupations and work: for example sketching, playing golf or a musical instrument, or arts and crafts in general are, for some, the means of earning a living, while for others, they are leisure. To qualify as leisure, an activity must be one we choose to pursue within the free time available to us. Leisure also implies a state of mind in which feelings of well-being are to the fore. Taking account of these concepts, Ravetz (1984) has offered the following definition:

Leisure is time left over from work when a person involves himself in activity, or non-activity, of his own free will, for pleasure and not for remuneration, and enjoys a feeling of well-being, relaxation or stimulation.

A possible flaw in this definition is its assumption that leisure is 'time left over from work'. The implications of this kind of assumption will be considered in due course. However, a number of influential theorists do contend that leisure is only amenable to analysis insofar as it relates to paid work.

Work and leisure

Although leisure is not necessarily the opposite of work, a great deal of sociological research has examined the relationship between them. The influence of occupational status on leisure has been a popular theme. There appears to be some connection between socio-economic status and the use of leisure, but it is a loose one (Roberts 1974). People in similar jobs may have quite different interests, and some leisure activities – such as watching television and reading newspapers – are common to all social groups.

Parker (1971) has attempted to identify broad trends. He suggests that people tend to use their leisure in one of three ways:

- as an *extension* of work
- as the *opposite* of work
- as *complementary* to work.

In the extension pattern, there is not much difference between the individual's behaviour at or away from work. Free time is spent 'talking shop' or building up skills and information that are relevant to work. Professional people and those whose occupations are intrinsically satisfying are more likely to be found in the extension category. Individuals whose jobs are repetitive and physically demanding (e.g. coal-miners) tend to view leisure as the opposite of work. They enjoy their free time more than their work, and see it as providing compensation and release; leisure activities are quite distinct from those that relate to the job. The complementary pattern involves striking a more even balance between work and leisure, participation in each area of life being relatively passive.

This pattern tends to typify office clerks and those whose jobs are neither particularly challenging nor downright disagreeable. For this group, work has little impact (positive or negative) on the business of leisure.

Parker's analysis is not without interest, but it remains an analysis of trends. The relationship between job status and leisure is not yet established to the extent that we can predict a person's leisure activities on the basis of his or her job with any real degree of precision. Nor can it necessarily be assumed that when a person is fortunate enough to have access to both domains, it is always work that determines the nature of leisure. Individuals who place a high value on leisure may choose undemanding jobs that do not divert their energies from this sphere; or they may choose jobs simply on the grounds that they finance their preferred leisure pursuits. Roberts (1974) has pointed out that choices in either field reflect a person's value system. Thus, the presumed cause and effect relationship may well be spurious.

The concept of fusion

It has already been acknowledged that leisure cannot be distinguished from work on the basis of activity alone. Historically, work and leisure merged in hunting and farming occupations, and this type of fusion has its modern counterpart: coffee and lunch breaks, business conferences and staff outings are contemporary instances of fusion.

It is clear that, in view of fusion, leisure cannot adequately be defined in terms of an inverse relation to work. Such definitions have disadvantages in addition to inconsistency, notably their negative connotations. Whereas today, the notion of 'fun morality' is gaining ground, leisure juxtaposed with work traditionally implied a sense of guilt. Thus, Margaret Mead (1957) wrote that unearned leisure was a vice that would have to be paid for later. It is, of course, doubtful that leisure has to be 'earned' in the first place. Many people have never worked, in the sense of engaging in paid employment. Obviously such people have a great deal of free time, but this is not to say they have leisure time (see below).

Leisure and the use of free time

Free time is a prerequisite for leisure, yet there are people who complain at having too much time on their hands. Some people feel guilty at this, or feel bored or depressed, or take a second job. Among those who contend that leisure is neither non-work nor the equivalent of free time, the strongest case has been made by de Grazia (1964; 1968). He argues that if leisure is viewed in relation to work, then time becomes split into job time and free time. Under these circumstances, time off work amounts at best to a period of rest or recreation. According to de Grazia, leisure is not a quantitative phenomenon, but a qualitative state which offers the benefits of cultivating a free mind. Only those who are liberated from work, social and financial pressures are really in a position to take advantage of leisure. De Grazia makes the point that not everyone has the temperament for leisure; for most people, it does not offer sufficient guidelines or sense of purpose. Thus, he suggests (de Grazia 1964) that leisure is 'a state of being, a condition of man, which few desire and fewer achieve'.

There appears to be wide agreement that the trend towards increased free time is likely to continue, whether this increase be forced or voluntary. It should be noted at this point that the concept of forced free time extends beyond non-job time imposed upon people by unemployment, illness and the like. It can also include vacation periods in which people feel obliged to enjoy their supposed leisure in fairly frenetic fashion. In view of the purported increase in free time – to which the rapid growth of the leisure industry bears witness – the argument has been made that our educational system has ill-prepared us to deal with this change. Modern education tends to be vocationally oriented, whereas de Grazia has argued that a liberal education best equips the person for leisure. While his views might appear extreme to many, few would disagree with the claim that some sort of education for leisure is desirable.

Occupational therapy recognises that leisure offers opportunities for social participation, creativity and growth in self-esteem. As Adolf Meyer pointed out early in the century, mental health requires a positive structuring of time and the development of habits appropriate to daily living (Meyer 1917). Leisure interests are ideally suited to promoting gains in these areas. Crafts and games also enhance cognitive functions, such as memory and concentration (Fig. 8.2(a) & (b)). Teaching the skills and activities required to enjoy leisure are an important part of the therapist's repertoire. However, as Nichol (1964) points out, the therapist must keep the issue of temporal adaptation in mind, and try to maintain a balance between the time patients spend on ADL, leisure and work-oriented activities.

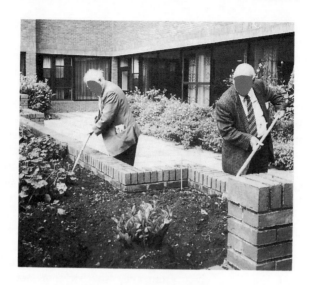

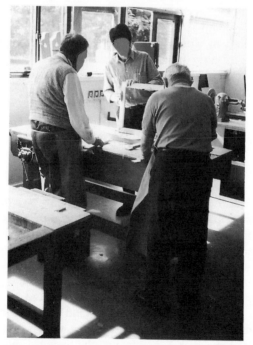

Fig. 8.2 Activities such as gardening and woodwork enhance physical function while offering greater ot lesser degrees of challenge in accordance with the goals of intervention. (Source: Lothian Health Board.)

RETIREMENT

As noted in our discussion of normal development, the mandatory age of retirement in most occupations is 65 years. Since some employees take early retirement, and some occupations do not have a mandatory retirement age, most people give up work at some point between the age of 60 and 70 years. Attitudes to the prospect vary widely. Some workers look forward to a well-earned rest, while others face the prospect with dread. Commonly expressed fears refer to living on a reduced income, loss of routine and lack of contact with colleagues. People in positions with high socio-economic status may dislike the prospect of losing authority and prestige. Geist (1968) notes that people are more likely to resist the idea of retirement before it actually takes place, and that anxiety tends to reach a peak as the individual comes close to retirement age. Once retirement has occurred, anxiety usually subsides and adjustment is often more favourable than anticipated.

Adjustment to retirement

Studies of ageing and retirement have shown that there is no single pattern of successful adjustment. Reichard et al's (1962) classical study of retired individuals found three distinct personality types among a sample of elderly men who were considered to have adjusted well. In addition to a 'mature' realistic group – whom one would expect to fall into the category – passive, 'rocking-chair' types, and 'armoured' defensively active types had also successfully adapted to the ageing process, each in their own fashion. Poorly adjusted men tended to be angry and resentful. They blamed other people for the failures and disappointments of their lives, or else turned their resentment inwards. There is no evidence to indicate discontinuity between middle- and late adulthood. In general, there is a great deal of consistency between patterns of adjustment in early life and adjustment after retirement. The mature and active groups studied by Reichard each continued to involve themselves in social and organisational activities and maintained a range of hobbies (Fig. 8.3).

Atchley (1976) has proposed a number of retirement phases. *Remote* and *near* phases precede the event, and retirement is followed by a *honeymoon* phase during which people exult in the novelty of spare time. This is a period wherein individuals catch up on all the things they wanted, but never had time, to do. The

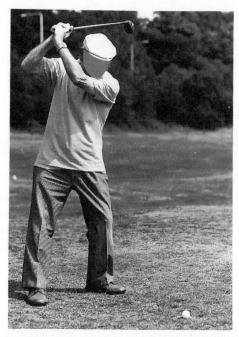

Fig. 8.3 Happily-retired people are much more likely to have hobbies than those who are unhappy. However, these hobbies are seldom newly discovered, tending to have been developed in earlier years (Geist 1968) (photograph reproduced from McClymont M et al 1991 Health visiting and elderly people, 2nd edn. Churchill Livingstone, Edinburgh by kind permission of Michael J. Denham).

honeymoon period draws to an end as routine sets in and, for some individuals, a *disenchantment* phase follows. This may involve a degree of depression, but in the ensuing *reorientation* and *stability* phases, realistic decisions about life-style are made, and the person becomes more self sufficient. The *termination* phase of retirement is marked by decreasing autonomy and, eventually, dependence on others. The study of Ekerdt et al (1985) has lent support to the idea that retirement is followed by a honeymoon phase that does not endure. Using questionnaire measures of life satisfaction, they found that recently retired males expressed higher levels of satisfaction than those retired for longer.

Although it is possible to lead a 'rocking-chair' life in retirement and yet be well-adapted, most investigators have found that people who are active when retired are better adjusted than those who are passive, and that they also report themselves more satisfied. The benefits of activity are not always acknowledged by staff who care for the 5% or so of retired individuals who live in residential accommodation. Slater (1984) observes that staff often encourage dependency in the elderly to save their own time and energy, especially where mobility is a problem. Staff and residents may subscribe equally to the principle of least effort but, as he remarks:

> . . . such an apparently reasonable arrangement ultimately leads to a model of residents as 'objects' to be 'serviced', to situations where independence and autonomy are undermined and where social interaction – the mainstay of a humane model of man – is marked by its absence.
>
> (Slater 1984, p 348)

Pre-retirement planning

It has frequently been suggested (e.g. Havighurst 1982) that the retirement process should be made more flexible so as to cater better for the variety of needs that characterise people over the age of 60. Suggestions include a less stringent approach to compulsory retirement and a gradual decrease in working hours instead of abrupt cessation. Pre-retirement planning on a wider scale has also been advocated, particularly for those who are apprehensive at the prospect of ceasing work. A growing number of companies are sponsoring pre-retirement policies, which offer counselling services and can advise on financial provision for the future, leisure and alternative work opportunities, further education and the like. De Grazia has suggested that retired individuals are more likely than other groups in modern society to profit from their free time to the extent that it can constitute leisure. Most have financial resources of some kind, however meagre, and because free time is not merely rest time, slotted between periods of work, retired people are perfectly positioned to cultivate the frame of mind appropriate to leisure. Geist (1968) focused on leisure activities as indices of well-being in retirement, pointing out that those who most enjoy this particular phase of life are those who have had durable hobbies of a kind that leisure can satisfy. Having reviewed the literature, he concludes that well-adjusted retired people are more likely than the maladjusted to travel and make excursions, pursue education, cultivate intellectual or artistic skills, and engage in productive hobbies, such as carpentry or gardening.

9. Changing approaches to health care

TRADITIONS OF CARE

The history of care has always been one in which a number of diverse approaches have co-existed, at times uneasily. This diversity was especially evident during the nineteenth century. That century saw a vast increase in the number of orphanages, schools, workhouses, asylums and hospitals built specifically to cater for the most deprived members of society. Some of these institutions were state-controlled, and some established and controlled by religious charities or other voluntary bodies. Alongside these developments, there also existed informal approaches to welfare. Some landlords and employers were aware of their obligations to their tenants and employees, and looked after their needs in a spirit of paternalistic benevolence. However, these obligations were not copper-fastened by statute, and horrific instances of exploitation were widespread, especially during the industrial revolution. As today, support systems also included help provided by nuclear and extended families, and by friends, neighbours and wider kin.

During the early decades of the nineteenth century, there was scant recognition of the need for government intervention in the social system. In the United Kingdom, the Poor Law, and in particular the Poor Law Report of 1834, did acknowledge the need for a degree of intervention, but it involved applying stringent means-test-based criteria to decisions about who should benefit from the very basic services offered. Because access to public support systems was not seen as a universal right, assistance under the Poor Law tended to carry with it a social stigma and connotations of charity, that were retained in the public mind for over a century. Nevertheless, the law did inspire public bodies and private charities to unite in efforts to build structures that would cater for the needs of the 'deserving poor'.

These nineteenth and early twentieth century reforms were, of course, implemented in the context of 'laissez-faire' liberal philosophy (Jordan 1976). The economists and politicians who espoused this philosophy were committed to policies of state intervention where these were clearly necessary to reduce inequalities. However, apart from introducing progressive taxation and limited policies of insurance, they did not agree with large-scale intervention programmes. The prevailing belief was that scientific and commercial advance would generate the prosperity necessary to remedy most social evils; it was further believed that government interference in economic matters would slow down the pace of progress and, in the long run, impede social reform – hence the proliferation of institutions whose services were offered to restricted sections of the population. However, following World War II, the concept that the state should provide health and educational services for everyone gained ground, inspired largely by the economic philosophies of Karl Marx and John Maynard Keynes. In Britain, the National Assistance Act of 1948 saw the final demise of the Poor Law, and country after country became increasingly committed to the idea of state responsibility for welfare.

RESIDENTIAL CARE

Developments during the nineteenth century reflected demands for a greater variety of institutions, so as to improve the quality of care offered, particularly to the young. During the 1840s, hundreds of juvenile offenders were committed annually to adult gaols, where they frequently fell under the malign influence of hardened long-term prisoners. In the wake of recognition that provisions for children were woefully inadequate, in this and other respects, reformatories and industrial schools were built after the 1850s as alternatives to prison. These were superseded in turn by approved schools and, later still, by community homes for the young (Clough 1982). The 1870s saw a further proliferation of homes for orphaned and abandoned children, and this continued for several decades. Inspired by pioneers such as Dr Barnado, these homes aimed at the very least to provide food, shelter and the basic necessities of life.

The tendency to respond to social problems by building yet more institutions continued until comparatively recently. Following the establishment of residential centres for children, similar provisions were made for the handicapped, the mentally ill and the elderly.

Clough (1981) reports that between 1959 and 1973, the number of residents in local authority old people's homes grew from 60 900 to 100 400. At the same time, there was a dramatic change in the type of accommodation provided. Whereas in 1959 most of the residents lived in large homes (those with 70 or more places), only 12% did so in 1973, reflecting a marked swing to medium-sized units. These changes were due to growing objections to large-scale institutions (see below). Nevertheless, despite these objections, demands for residential care continued during the 1970s. Brearley (1982) reports that in 1978 over 100 000 children were in care in England and Wales, and that 40 000 of these were placed in some kind of residential accommodation. In the same year, figures for the United Kingdom show that the average *daily* number of bed users in psychiatric hospitals was 102 700, while almost 170 000 elderly people lived in residential accommodation provided by local authority, voluntary and private bodies. (Central Statistical Office 1981). While demand for residential facilities remained strong during the 1980s, resources were increasingly devoted to alternative services.

Disadvantages of institutional living

Even as institutions mushroomed during the Victorian era, they were not without their critics. The novels of Charles Dickens and Charlotte Brontë, among others, often portrayed the harsh realities of life in Victorian orphanages and charity schools. While residential centres for children followed more enlightened policies in the twentieth century, researchers have pointed out that, in the early decades, they were primarily concerned with hygiene, efficiency and serving the physical needs of those in their care. In a number of publications dating from the early 1950s (e.g. Bowlby 1953), Bowlby has insisted that institutions are ill-equipped to meet children's emotional needs. He drew attention to the fact that staff rota systems, staff turnover, and the sheer numbers of children in any one building made it impossible for children to establish close emotional ties with their carers. Bowlby claimed that children reared in large institutions are at risk of irreparable emotional and intellectual damage, and contended that many such children develop a psychopathic 'affectionless' character which inclines them to crime in adolescence. On the grounds that 'mother-love' and bonding with a mother-figure in infancy are essential for normal emotional development, he concluded that family care, no matter how deficient it might be, is preferable to confinement in an institution.

Following concern about standards in children's homes voiced in the Curtis Committee report of 1946, and following confirmation of Bowlby's findings by a number of other investigators in Europe and North America, facilities for children in care changed dramatically. Homes became smaller and organised along the lines of the natural family, with house parents caring for a small, intimate group. The ideal today is that children in family-type homes should participate as fully as possible in community life; that they should join local libraries, clubs and sports centres, take part in community activities, visit other children and have them back home on return visits.

The trend away from large, impersonal institutions is also evident, as noted above, in the building of new homes for the elderly. Increasingly, these comprise small units, built around a central large unit, in which assistance from nursing and other staff is available as necessary. Maximum independence in self-care is encouraged and, indeed, residential care is no longer the preferred option. Community-care policies are oriented to providing support services to the elderly in their own homes as far as is reasonably possible.

Mental disorder and institutionalisation

Perhaps the most serious indictment of institutions has come from critics of traditional psychiatric hospitals. As noted in Chapter 2, Laing, Szasz and others (e.g. Cooper 1967) have challenged the assumption that mental 'illness' is comparable to physical illness and, accordingly, have condemned treatment methods based on this assumption. Yet, despite the fact that psychiatric procedures are open to severe criticism, innovations in drug therapy have undeniable advantages. The advent of new psychotropic drugs in the mid-1950s allowed doctors to control the more extreme manifestations of psychological problems, thereby facilitating early release from hospital. In place of long-term residence, patients could now return to the community, although this tended to be on a 'revolving door' basis, characterised by cycles of admission, release and readmission. Investigators were now ready to investigate the effectiveness of institutions in preparing patients to face the outside world.

Goffman

Early twentieth century hospitals stressed the custodial over the treatment aspect of care, and saw their role as one of relieving society of its burden of responsibility for mental deviants. Conditions in these asylums were far from favourable, and Deutsch's 'Shame of the States' (1948) drew attention to the cruel and appalling conditions that prevailed in many state hospitals. Goffman's subsequent studies took place against a background of early debate about the nature of mental disorder and in the context of newer treatment methods. Yet he paid scant attention to these issues. His concern was with the effects of institutions on the health and autonomy of inmates. In his book *Asylums* (1961), Goffman maintained that mental hospitals are 'total institutions' which engulf their inhabitants. On admission, the individual acquires the status of a patient, and maintains this sick role in order to adapt to the unique and isolated culture that surrounds him; likewise, he accepts the power that staff have over his actions. In the process, his sense of self is destroyed and he experiences 'disculturation' whereby his capacity to manage social relationships in the outside world is diminished. Goffman contends that institutional residence tends to worsen the condition for which a patient was originally admitted.

Barton

Barton (1966) identified several features of the institutional environment which contribute to what Goffman has described as 'profanations of self'. Inhabitants are alienated from the external world and may receive few visits from relatives because of the stigma attached to their situation. Staff are usually authoritative and may dictate minute details of a person's life, such as what clothes to wear, or when to go to bed. Efforts by patients to engage in autonomous behaviour may disrupt routine and are likely to be discouraged. The individual is without personal friends; possessions are communal and events impersonal. According to Barton, these conditions lead to 'institutional neurosis' entailing apathy, lack of initiative, submissiveness and loss of interest in the future.

Response to the problem of 'institutionalisation'

Goffman and Barton were writing about state mental hospitals in the 1950s and at the dawn of the 1960s, and although their claims are not generalisable, they were sufficiently plausible and dramatic to alert health professionals to the dangers of what is now termed 'institutionalisation'. This term is used to characterise the response to long-term custodial care. It indicates that when people are relieved of the responsibility of managing their own lives, they develop a disorder over and above that for which they were originally admitted. The chief characteristics of institutionalisation are: apathy, dependency on caregivers, no expression of resentment at unfair treatment, loss of individuality and of interest in decision-making, and helplessness. It is frequently seen among mental hospital inmates and among the elderly in residential care and tends to be related to length of stay. Scrutiny of the institutions studied further revealed that, in many cases, disabled and elderly people were placed in homes for those with a mental disability for the simple reason that there was nowhere else for them to go – a practice which still continues in countries whose economies are relatively underdeveloped. The concept of 'institutionalisation' highlighted the need for more occupational therapists and more professionals whose remedial policies espouse humanistic values. However, the status and scope of alternative treatment philosophies still depends on the extent to which they can be accommodated to the dominant medical model within hospitals, and on whether they receive patronage from medical personnel (Goldie 1977, Black 1982).

The radical-psychiatry argument that treatment procedures can constitute forms of violence against the person, and that compulsory detention is a violation of human rights has, despite its controversial nature, made an impact. Since the eighties, there have been legal constraints in the United Kingdom on admitting people to institutions and detaining them there against their will; and those constraints have their counterparts in other countries. The goal of closing down Victorian asylums and replacing them with community-based services is a long-standing one, but one that so far has met with mixed success. The Government White Paper, 'Better services for the mentally ill' (DHSS 1975) accepted that expectations during the early sixties of halving the psychiatric hospital population were not as yet fulfilled, but it reiterated the general aim of achieving 'a shift in the balance between hospital and social services care'.

COMMUNITY CARE

A government document on priorities for the Health and Social Services (DHSS 1981a: 21) stated that a major objective for many years had been to foster community care for the main client groups – the elderly, mentally ill and handicapped people, disabled people, and children – and that 'the general aim is to maintain a person's link with family and friends and normal life, and to offer the support that meets his or her particular needs'. The principles and objectives of community care were later stated more fully in evidence given to the House of Commons Committee on Social Services in 1985 (HC 13 1984–1985; Box 9.1).

Box 9.1   The principles and objectives of community care (DHSS 1985)

- to enable an individual to remain in his own home wherever possible rather than being cared for in a hospital or residential home
- to give support and relief to informal carers (family, friends and neighbours) coping with the stress of caring for a dependent person
- to deliver appropriate help, by the means which cause the least possible disruption to ordinary living
- to relieve the stresses and strains contributing to or arising from physical or emotional disorder
- to provide the most cost-effective package of services to meet the needs and wishes of those being helped
- to integrate all the resources of a geographical area in order to support the individuals within it.

Smaller residential units

Brearley (1982) writes that the term 'community care' is generally used to distinguish residential from non-residential provisions, and that pronouncements on the subject typically view residential care in an unfavourable light, usually as a last resort. He contends that this view bears upon the low morale and status of residential workers, and that it frequently contributes to feelings of professional isolation. The majority of objections to residential centres have, however, concentrated on very large, highly regimented institutions. The trend towards smaller units, sheltered homes and hostels continues, therefore, alongside the development of day-care facilities.

When proposals for community care were first put forward, they were welcomed on humanitarian grounds and in the expectation that they would produce considerable economies. Wherever Victorian institutions have been restored and re-equipped, the costs involved have been enormous. However, the provision of smaller units is not an inexpensive option. For example, Clough (1982) points out that it is not axiomatic that small family-style residences for children are more viable than their predecessors, economically or otherwise. These can be difficult to finance and staff, and have been questioned 'because of the artificiality of a "home" pretending to be like any other family'. Clough notes that, in spite of attempts to expand fostering, the number of children and young people in residential care increased during the 1970s and early 1980s.

Mental disability

Perhaps the most serious problem facing providers of care in the 1990s is that of meeting the needs of persons with a mental disability. Closure of the older Victorian-style institutions has created a shortage of accommodation, and the 1983 reforms of the Mental Health Act have made it more difficult to admit and detain a person compulsorily. Arguably, the provision of alternative services has not kept pace with the enthusiasm for closure. In the United Kingdom, the media have frequently drawn attention to the plight of parents whose adult, and sometimes violent, offspring are desperately in need of acute admission, but who cannot gain access to hospital for legal reasons, for lack of bed-space or because of reluctance on the part of doctors to take away a person's liberty. Thus, many writers and broadcasters, (e.g. Wallace 1988) suggest that the pendulum has swung too far. There remain cases, too, of patients discharged to hopelessly inadequate accommodation, and instances of those who simply cannot cope with the material demands of daily life; this situation has prompted Lapping (1974) to suggest that the term 'community careless' may be the more appropriate one.

It seems clear that, while the intentions behind the move towards community care are humane and praiseworthy, the utopian vision of a caring community, receptive to everyone in need, is not easy to achieve. Those charged with the responsibility of planning services must keep in mind the goal of achieving an appropriate balance of facilities, which serve the best interests of those for whom they are designed. Above all, there is a need for fully thought-out and practical policies of after-care.

Provision for the disabled in the European Community

The European Community recognises that wide differences exist among member states in resources devoted to caring for the handicapped, and in criteria for defining disabled groups. For purposes of joint action, the Council of Ministers in 1974 defined a handicap as 'any limitation of a person's physical or mental ability which affects his daily activity and his work . . .'. The Community is fully committed to equality, integration, and community care for persons with a disability but, given the diverging approaches to the problem by the countries concerned, it has, for practical reasons, given priority to the issue of rehabilitation. To date, hundreds of millions of pounds have been spent on vocational training and rehabilitation programmes through the auspices of the European Social Fund. There remains the difficulty (Clarke 1990) that, for many disabled persons, training for a job in the open work-force, or even in sheltered employment, is not a realistic option. For these, there is an urgent need for alternative support systems, including day-centres. In smaller European countries, for example Ireland, it is easy to keep track of the number of centres available to those who need them, but less easy to compile statistics on the number of persons in need, due chiefly to limited resources. Day-activity and day-care centres expanded rapidly in Ireland during the 1980s, and there are currently 156 of these throughout the country. As the journal of the National Rehabilitation Board illustrates *, in Ireland, day centres for people with mental illness are most common, followed by those for people with mental handicap. There are fewer for those with mixed handicaps, and a relative shortage of centres (8% of the total) for people with physical handicap. As Clarke (1990) notes 'There are very few statistics relating to physically disabled people in Ireland – a situation which does not assist in the planning and development of appropriate services'.

Inconsistencies of information and strategies between member states depict some of the problems faced by the European Community, as it is extremely difficult to implement desirable programmes in the absence of clear-cut data and guidelines. Although the

---

* Slanuacht: the Journal of the National Rehabilitation Board, May 1990.

Community does plan to increase its financial input into research, education for handicapped children, employment facilities and many other areas, there are numerous obstacles to progress. Meanwhile, firm and comprehensive policies are needed at national levels.

Community care in the United Kingdom: Government proposals

Towards the end of the 1980s, two important government documents addressed the issue of community care: the Griffiths Report, 'Community care: agenda for action' in 1988, and the 1989 White Paper 'Caring for people: community care in the next decade and beyond'.

The terms of reference for the Griffiths Report concentrated on current use of funds in supporting community care policy, and on recommendations as to how funds might be used to contribute to a more effective service. The Report suggested that local authority social services should have primary responsibility for assessing individual needs, and for designing and delivering care arrangements. It was claimed that an overlap of roles (for example between public housing and social service authorities) limits efficiency and creates confusion, and that the issue of responsibility is crucial. The Report therefore proposed the appointment of a Minister of State in the *DHSS* who would be clearly identified as being responsible for community care. In addition, the Report accepted that problems of responsibility for after-care arise from closure of large mental hospitals. It recommended that a clear package of care be devised for each discharged person and that its management be supervised, and support provided, by one individual, named carer.

In the White Paper of 1989, the Government reiterated its commitment to community care and to the principle of allotting responsibility, in the areas mentioned by Griffiths, to local authorities. Government proposals included the suggestion that local authorities produce and publish clear plans for the delivery of community services, and that they liaise with health authorities and the independent sector in devising these plans. The White Paper further proposed that carers should have the practical support necessary to them in their work, and 1990 saw the provision of new financial allowances for 'informal' care givers.

Prior to the publication of the documents outlined above, the Audit Commission Report ('Making a reality of community care',

December 1986) had suggested that changing approaches to care necessarily have implications for the supply and training of personnel. The Commission recommended that assistant carers in a number of roles should be united in a new occupational category of 'community carers'. The Griffiths Report notes that the creation of such a category would require definition and review of the training needs involved. It adds that, in view of new responsibilities proposed for local authorities, training systems for professional staff will need to give greater emphasis to management skills.

THE IMPLICATIONS OF CHANGE FOR OCCUPATIONAL THERAPY

Towards the end of the 1980s, the College of Occupational Therapists commissioned an independent report on the existing state and future role of occupational therapy in the United Kingdom. The commission, whose members came from disparate disciplines, had as chairman Louis Blom-Cooper QC, and it produced its report, entitled 'Occupational therapy: an emerging profession in health care' in 1989 (Blom-Cooper 1989). The Report noted that the establishment and maintenance of professional identity and autonomy remain problems facing occupational therapists, and suggested several reasons for this situation. These include (1) the dominant position of medical personnel in the health service, and of social workers in local authority social services; and (2) stereotyping of the profession and its pronounced female composition. Stereotyping reflects a distorted and grossly oversimplified view of professional activities. The related problem of perceived low professional status is compounded by the preponderance of women in the field. The Report noted that the dominant role of the medical and social work professions affects the division of labour in health care. It likewise affects the autonomy of occupational therapists, who must court the more dominant professions for patronage and for access to clients, and who may have to yield to their authority where there is apparent conflict of professional objectives.

On the issue of the profession's future role and identity, the Commission surmised that budgetary restrictions will have implications for occupational therapists, one way or another: it may be 'seen as peripheral to the main medical and surgical objectives of cure' or there may be efforts:

to find ways of substituting pseudo-occupational therapy, performed by other professional groups or by technical assistants with no qualification in occupational therapy as such, in poor substitution for the genuine article. There is even talk in responsible circles of ending the separate identity of the various professions within the general field of rehabilitation and creating a single profession with specialisms developing only after initial training.

(Blom-Cooper 1989, pp 20–21)

Rehabilitation professions

The Commission considered that the prospect of a watered-down version of occupational therapy as a suggested solution to shortages of resources paradoxically reflects the profession's success over recent decades. The profession is expanding rapidly, demand for its services far exceeds supply, and a high drop-out rate prevails. Among districts responding to the Commission's enquiry, almost 1500 positions were left unfilled at the end of March 1988. On a national scale, this represents 10.3% of posts funded in the NHS and 11.9% of local authority funded posts. The Commission estimated that by the end of the century, an 80% expansion in the number of qualified occupational therapists will be required to meet demand. It did not accept that a generalist rehabilitation profession should replace the specialist professions that now exist – at least in the immediate future. However, the Commission did recommend that the possibility of joining forces with physiotherapy – to form a single profession that provided for post-qualification specialisation – receive serious consideration, and that, in the long run, a united profession of rehabilitation therapists might be desirable. These issues should, therefore, be kept under review. The Commission further suggested that opportunities for systematic training should be offered to Helpers and Technical Instructors, and that those who receive such training be given appropriate recognition. The Commission also recommended the adoption of procedures to ensure that untrained staff are not left to undertake therapeutic work for which they are not prepared. It suggested, too, (p 88) that claims to professional status would be enhanced 'by devising ways of measuring and monitoring the effectiveness and efficiency of practices, procedures and organisational arrangements'.

Redeployment to community care sector

In the context of community care, the Commission of Inquiry stressed that the pace of relocation from hospital to community must be accelerated. At the time of writing of the Report (June 1989), the preponderance of occupational therapists in the hospital sector was 80%, as against 20% deployed in the community care sector. While recognising that redeployment will inevitably involve some problems, the Commission urged occupational therapists to prepare themselves for new opportunities, and for an exciting future in which occupational therapy will cease to be a 'submerged profession'.

The future and its challenges

Although long-term institutional care has received a bad press in recent decades, it has in the past served several useful functions. Many inhabitants valued the routine and security offered, and the friendships formed. Residences also became second homes for children with relatively severe handicaps, whose families found that the burden of minding them imposed too great a strain. In the future, admission to residential care will be even rarer than it is at present, and duration of stay probably shorter. In these circumstances, the need for health professionals to teach daily-living skills will be ever more acute. People admitted to short-term residential care will need help to face the daily management problems associated with early release. For the growing numbers receiving community care, the teaching of work, leisure and daily-living activities is of invaluable benefit not only to the individuals in question, but also to their families, who can no longer depend on institutional support systems. Occupational therapists must try to meet the growing demand for their skills in a setting whose structures and hierarchy of authority will be less rigid than those which currently prevail, and respond to the challenges of the future in a context of greater autonomy.

Conclusions

As the 1989 Commission of Inquiry reported, the problems facing occupational therapy today result from the profession's successes, and not its failures, the main problem being that there are simply not enough occupational therapists available to meet current and future requirements. It is primarily this shortfall in personnel that has inspired recommendations to introduce new categories of less skilled carers. Whatever doubts occupational therapists may have about their own status, there is statistical evidence that health and social services rely upon their expertise to maximise the independence, competence and dignity of those in need of help.

References

CHAPTER 1

Allport G W 1963 Pattern and growth in personality. Holt, Rinehart and Winston, New York

AOTA Representative Assembly Minutes 1981 American Journal of Occupational Therapy 13: 792–802

Asch S E 1952 Social psychology. Prentice-Hall, Englewood Cliff, New Jersey

Asch SE 1955 Opinions and social pressures. Scientific American 193: 31–35

Bell D 1973 The coming of the post-industrial society: a venture in social forecasting. Basic Books, New York

Chorley R J, Haggett P 1967 Models in geography. Methuen, London

Clark P N 1979 Human development through occupation: Theoretical frameworks in contemporary occupational therapy practice. Part one. American Journal of Occupational Therapy 33 (8): 504–514

Evans J D 1985 Invitation to psychological research. Holt, Rinehart and Winston, New York

Hawking S W 1988 A brief history of time. Bantam Press, London

Kielhofner G (ed) 1985 A model of human occupation: theory and application. Williams and Wilkins, Baltimore

Kuhn T S 1962 The structure of scientific revolutions. University of Chicago Press, Chicago (Revised edn, 1969)

Kuhn T S 1977 The essential tension: selected studies on scientific tradition and change. University of Chicago Press, Chicago

Lakatos I 1970 Falsification and the methodology of scientific research programmes. In: Lakatos I, Musgrave A (eds) Criticism and the growth of knowledge. Cambridge University Press, Cambridge

Lipsey R G 1983 An introduction to positive economics. Weidenfeld and Nicolson, London

Magee B 1973 Popper. Fontana, London

Mocellin G 1984 Adaptation, coping and competence? Theoretical choice and professional decisions in occupational therapy. Proceedings of the Australian Association of Occupational Therapists 2

Mosey A C 1970 Three frames of reference for mental health. Charles B. Slack, Thorofare, New Jersey

Mosey A C 1981 Occupational therapy: configuration of a profession. Raven Press, New York

Popper K 1959 The logic of scientific discovery. Hutchinson, London

Popper K 1966 The open society and its enemies. Routledge and Kegan Paul, London

Popper K 1966 Unended quest: an intellectual autobiography Fontana/Collins, Glasgow

Popper K 1970 Normal science and its dangers. In: Lakatos I, A Musgrave (eds) Criticism and the growth of knowledge. Cambridge University Press, Cambridge

Reed K L, Sanderson S (1983) Concepts of occupational therapy. Williams and Wilkins, Baltimore

Turner A 1981 The practice of occupational therapy: an introduction to the treatment of physical dysfunction. Churchill Livingstone, Edinburgh

Watson J 1968 The double helix. Weidenfeld and Nicolson, London

CHAPTER 2

Barris R, Kielhofner G, Watts J 1983 Psychosocial occupational therapy: practice in a pluralistic arena. Ramsco, Laurel, Maryland

Beck A T 1962 Reliability of psychiatry 119: 210–216

Browne I 1990 R D Laing and the challenge to psychiatry. The Irish Times, April 25th, p 9

Capra F 1983 The turning point: Science, society and the rising culture. Fontana (Flamingo), London

Coleman V 1988 The health scandal: your health in crisis. Sidgwick and Jackson, London

Cracknell E 1984 Humanistic psychology. In: Willson M (ed) Occupational therapy in short-term psychiatry. Churchill Livingstone, Edinburgh

Davison G C, Neale J M 1986 Abnormal psychology, 4th edn. Wiley, New York

Fontana A 1966 Familial etiology of schizophrenia. Is a scientific methodology possible? Psychological Bulletin 66: 214–228

Friedhoff A J, van Winkle E 1962 Isolation and characterization of a compound from the urine of schizophrenics. Nature 194: 897

Goldstein M J 1985 The UCLA family project. Paper presented at the High Risk Consortium Conference, April, San Francisco

Goldstein M J, Rodnick E 1975 The family's contribution to the etiology of schizophrenia: current status. Schizophrenia Bulletin 14: 48–63

Gottesman I, Shields J 1982 Schizophrenia: the epigenetic puzzle. Cambridge University Press, New York

Greenblatt M, Myerson P G 1949 Medical progress, psychosurgery. New England Journal of Medicine 240: 1006–1007

Heston L L 1966 Psychiatric disorders in foster home reared children of schizophrenic mothers. British Journal of Psychiatry 112: 819–825

Illich I 1976 Medical nemesis: the expropriation of health. Pantheon Books, New York

Kallman F J 1958 The use of genetics in psychiatry. Journal of Mental Science 104: 542–549

Kammen D P, van Bunney W E, Docherty J P et al 1977 Amphetamine-induced catecholamine activation in schizophrenia and depression. Advances in Biochemical Psychopharmacology 16: 655–659

Kielhofner G, Burke J P 1983 The evolution of knowledge and practice in occupational therapy: past, present and future. In: Kielhofner (ed) Health through occupation: theory and practice in occupational therapy. F A Davis, Philadelphia

Kielhofner G (ed) 1985 A model of human occupation: theory and application. Williams and Wilkins, Baltimore

Laing R D 1976 The facts of life. Penguin Books, London

Laing R D 1964 Is schizophrenia a disease? International Journal of Social Psychiatry 10: 184–193

Laing R D 1960 The divided self. Tavistock, London

Leff J P 1982 Schizophrenia and sensitivity to the family environment. Schizophrenia Bulletin 85: 716–726

Lidz T 1973 The origin and treatment of schizophrenic disorders. Basic Books, New York

Mackay D 1975 Clinical psychology: theory and therapy. Methuen, London

Maslow A H 1958 Toward a psychology of being, 2nd edn. Van Nostrand, Princeton

Maslow A H 1970 Motivation and personality, 2nd edn. Harper and Row, New York

Mocellin G 1984 Adaptation, coping and competence? Theoretical choice and professional decisions in occupational therapy. Proceedings of the Australian Association of Occupational Therapists 2

Mosey A C 1970 Three frames of reference for mental health. Charles B Slack, Thorofare, NJ

Norton J P 1982 Expressed emotion, affective style, voice tone and communicated deviance as predictors of offspring schizophrenia spectrum disorders. Unpublished doctoral dissertation: UCLA (cited in Davison & Neale 1986)

Piaget J 1950 The pyschology of intelligence. Routledge, London

Rosenhahn D L 1973 On being sane in insane places. Science 179: 250–258

Rogers C R 1965 Client-centred therapy. Houghton, New York

Schmidt HO, Fonda C 1956 The reliability of psychiatric diagnosis. Journal of Abnormal and Social Psychology 52: 262–267

Sim M 1968 Guide to psychiatry. E & S Livingstone, Edinburgh, London

Singer M, Wynne L C 1963 Differentiating characteristics of the parents of childhood schizophrenics. American Journal of Psychiatry 120: 113–115

Skrabanek P, McCormick J 1989 Follies and fallacies in medicine. The Tarragon Press, Glasgow

Snyder S H 1980 Biological aspects of mental disorder. Oxford University Press, New York

Strauss J S 1982 Behavioral aspects of being disadvantaged and risk for schizophrenia. In: Parron DL, Solomon F, Jenkins CD (eds) Behavior, health, risks and social disadvantage. National Academy Press, Washington DC

Szasz T S 1960 The myth of mental illness. American Psychologist 15: 113–118

Weinberger D R, Wagner R L, Wyatt R J 1983 Neuropathological studies of schizophrenia: a selective review. Schizophrenia Bulletin 9: 193–212

CHAPTER 3

Allen C K 1985 Measurement and management of cognitive disabilities. Little, Brown, Boston

Allen C K 1985 Occupational therapy for psychiatric diseases. Little, Brown, Boston

AOTA Representative Assembly 1979 American Journal of Occupational Therapy 33: 785

Buckoven J S 1971 Legacy of moral treatment, 1800s to 1910. American Journal of Occupational Therapy

Clark P N 1979 Theoretical frameworks in contemporary occupational therapy practice, part 1. American Journal of Occupational Therapy 33: 509

Craig G J 1976 Human development. Prentice Hall, Englewood Cliffs, NJ pp 11, 12, 32

Engelhardt H T 1974 The concepts of health and disease. In: Spicher S F (ed) Evaluation and explanation in the biomedical sciences. Reidell, Dordrocht, Holland

Engelhardt H T 1977 Defining occupational therapy: the meaning of therapy and the virtues of occupation. American Journal of Occupational Therapy

Engelhardt H T 1986 The importance of values in shaping professional directions and behaviour. In: Target 2000, American Occupational Therapists' Association

European Community 1989 Proceedings of committee on occupational therapy.

Fidler G S 1969 The task oriented group as a context for treatment. American Journal of Occupational Therapy 23: 43–48

Heard C 1977 Occupational role acquisition: a perspective on the chronically disabled. American Journal of Occupation Therapy 31: 243–247

Hopkins H L 1988 Current basis for theory and philosophy of occupational therapy. In: Hopkins H L, Smith H D (eds) Williard and Spackman's Occupational therapy, 7th edn. JB Lippincott, Philadelphia, pp 38–42

Hopkins H L, Smith H D (eds) 1988 Williard and Spackman's Occupational therapy, 7th edn. Lippincott, Philadelphia

Kielhofner G 1977 Temporal adaptations. A conceptual framework for occupational therapy. American Journal of Occupational Therapy 31: 235

Kielhofner G, Burke J P 1982 The evolution of knowledge and practice in occupational therapy: past, present and future. In: Kielhofner G (ed). Health through occupation. FA Davis, Philadelphia

Kielhofner G, Burke J 1985 Components and determinants of human occupation. In: Kielhofner G (ed) 1985 A model of human occupation: theory and application. Williams and Wilkins, Baltimore

Korzybski A 1921 Manhood of humanity: the science and art of human engineering. Dutton, New York

Leuret F 1840 On the moral treatment of insanity. In: Licht S 1978 Occupational therapy. William and Wilkins, Baltimore

Licht S 1978 Occupational therapy source book. Williams and Wilkins, Baltimore

Llorens L A 1970 1969 Eleanor Clark Slagle lecture. American Journal of Occupational Therapy 24: 1–9

Llorens L A 1973 Activity analyses for cognitive-perceptual-motor dysfunction. American Journal of Occupational Therapy 27: 453

MacDonald M 1978 Occupational therapy in rehabilitation, 4th edn. Bailliere Tindall, London

Matsutsuyu J 1971 Occupational behaviour: a perspective on work and play. American Journal of Occupational Therapy 25: 291–294

Meyer A 1922 The philosophy of occupational therapy. Archives of Occupational therapy 1: 1–10

Mocellin G 1983 The use of activities in the treatment and rehabilitation of psychiatric patients: an overview. Australian Occupational Therapy Journal 29: 109–117

Mocellin 1984 Adaptation, coping or competence? Paper presented at Australian Association of Occupational Therapy, Perth, Western Australia

Mosey A C 1968 Recapitulation of ontogenesis: a theory for the practice of occupational therapy. American Journal of Occupational Therapy 22: 426–438

Mosey A C 1989 Occupational therapy. Configuration of a profession. Raven Press, New York

Proceedings of symposium of annual research, Occupational therapy, September, Washington University, St Louis, Missouri, USA

Reilly M 1966 A psychiatric occupational therapy programme as a teaching model. American Journal of Occupational Therapy 20: 61–67

Rogers J C 1982 Order and disorder in medicine and occupational therapy. American Journal of Occupational Therapy 36: 29–35

Siegler M, Osmond H 1974 Models of madness, models of medicine. Macmillan, New York

Skinner B F 1938 The behaviour of organisms. Appleton Century Croft, New York

West W L 1984 A reaffirmed philosophy and practice of occupational therapy for the 1980s. American Journal of Occupational Therapy 38: 15–23

White R W 1971 Motivation reconsidered: the concept of competence. Psychological Review 66(5): 297–333

Yerxa E J 1980 Audacious values: the energy source for occupational therapy practice. American Journal of Occupational Therapy 34

Yerxa E J 1980 Occupational therapy's role in creating a future climate of caring. American Journal of Occupational Therapy 34

CHAPTER 4

Allen C K 1985 Occupational therapy for psychiatric diseases: measurement and management of cognitive disabilities. Little Brown, Boston

Arlin P K 1975 Cognitive development in adulthood. A fifth stage? Developmental Psychology 11: 602–606

Arlin P K 1977 Piagetian operations in problem finding. Developmental Psychology 13: 297–298

Atchley R C 1976 The sociology of retirement. Schenkman, Cambridge Mass

Bender M P 1986 The neglect of the elderly by British psychologists. Bulletin of the British Psychological Society 39: 414–417

Bernstein B 1967 Social structure, language and learning. In: De Cecco J P (ed), The psychology of language, thought and instruction. Holt, Rinehart and Winston, New York

Bower T G R 1982 Development in infancy. W H Freeman, San Francisco

Bromley D B 1988 Human ageing. Penguin, Harmondsworth

Brown R 1973 A first language: the early stages. Harvard University Press, Cambridge, Mass

Cavanaugh J C 1983 Comprehension and retention of television programmes by 20- and 60-year olds. Journal of Gerontology 38(2): 190–196

Chomsky N 1965 Aspects of the theory of syntax. MIT Press, Cambridge, Mass

Colby A, Kohlberg L, Gibbs J, Lieberman M 1980 A longitudinal study of moral judgement. Unpublished manuscript: Harvard University.

Commons M L, Richards F A, Kuhn D 1982 Systematic and metasystematic reasoning: A case for levels of reasoning beyond Piaget's stage of formal operations. Child Development 53: 1058–1069

Costa P T, McCrae R R 1980 Still stable after all these years: personality as a key to some issues in aging. In: Baltes P B, Brim O G (eds) Life-span development and behavior 3. Academic Press, New York

Cumming E, Henry W 1961 Growing old. Basic Books, New York

Curtiss S 1977 Genie: a psycholinguistic study of a modern-day 'Wild Child'. Academic Press, New York

Davison G C, Neale J M 1986 Abnormal psychology. Wiley, New York

Donaldson M 1978 Children's minds. Fontana/Collins, London

Dyson J 1980 Sociopolitical influences on retirement research. Bulletin of the British Psychological Society 33: 128–130

Erikson E H 1963 Childhood and society, 2nd edn. Norton, New York

Erikson E H 1968 Identity: youth and crisis. Norton, New York

Fidler G S, Fidler J W 1963 Occupational therapy: A communication process in psychiatry. Macmillan, New York

Field D 1981 Can preschool children really learn to conserve? Child Development 52: 326–334

Flanagan J 1981 Some characteristics of 70-year-old workers. Paper presented at the annual meeting of the American Psychological Association.

Gelman R 1979 Preschool thought. American Psychologist 34: 900–904

Gesell A 1954 The ontogenesis of infant behaviour. In: Carmichael I (ed) Handbook of child psychology. Wiley, New York

Gould R L 1978 Transformations. Simon and Schuster, New York

Gruen G E 1965 Experiences affecting the development of number conservation in children. Child Development 36(4): 963–979

Harkins E B 1975 Effects of empty nest transition on self-report of psychological and physical well-being. Journal of Marriage and the Family 40: 549–556

Havighurst R J 1982 The world of work. In: Wolman BB (ed) Handbook of developmental psychology. Prentice Hall, Englewood Cliffs, New Jersey

Hopkins H L, Smith H D (eds) Williard and Spackman's Occupational therapy, 7th edn, section 2, p. 50. Lippincott, Philadelphia

Hughes F P, Noppe L D 1985 Human development across the life span. West, St Paul Minnesota

Hultsch D L 1971 Adult age differences in free classification and free recall. Developmental Psychology 4: 338–342

Hunt J M 1976 Ordinal scales of infant development and the nature of intelligence. In: Resnick LB (ed) The nature of intelligence. Lawrence Erlbaum, Hillsdale, New Jersey

Kielhofner G, Burke J 1985 Components and determinants of human occupation. In: Kielhofner G (ed) A model of human occupation: theory and application. Williams and Wilkins, Baltimore

Kohlberg L 1969 Stage and sequence. The cognitive developmental approach to socialization. In: Goslin D A (ed) Handbook of socialization theory and research. Rand McNally, Chicago

Labov W 1970 The study of nonstandard English. National Council of Teachers of English, Urbana, Illinois

Lenneberg E H 1967 Biological foundations of language. Wiley, New York

Levinson D J 1978 The seasons of a man's life. Ballantine, New York

Llorens L A 1970 1969 Eleanor Clark Slagle lecture. American Journal of Occupational Therapy 24: 1–9

Maddox G L 1964 Disengagement theory: a critical evaluation. The Gerontologist 4: 80–83

Maddox G L 1968 Persistence of life-style among the elderly. In: Neugarten B (ed) Middle age and ageing. University of Chicago Press, Chicago

Marcia J 1966 Development and validation of ego-identity status. Journal of Personality and Social Psychology 3: 551–558

Marcia J E 1980 Identity in adolescence. In: Adelson J (ed) Handbook of adolescent psychology. John Wiley, New York

May R B, Norton J M 1981 Training-task orders and transfer in conservation. Child Development 52: 904–913

Mindel C H, Vaughan C E 1978 A multidimensional approach to religiosity and disengagement. Journal of Gerontology 33: 103–108

Mosey A C 1981 Configuration of a profession. Raven Press, New York

Neimark E D 1979 Current status of formal operations research. Human Development 22: 60–67

Neugarten B L, Havighurst R J, Tobin S S 1968 Personality and patterns of aging. In: Neugarten B L (ed) Middle age and aging. Chicago University Press, Chicago

Neugarten B L 1970 Adaptation and the life cycle. Journal of Geriatric Psychiatry 136: 887–894

Offer D, Offer J B 1975 From teenage to young manhood: Basic Books, New York

Parten M B 1932 Social play among pre-school children. Journal of Abnormal Social Psychology 27: 243

Piaget J 1948 The origins of intelligence. Cook M (Trans). Illinois Free Press, Glencoe

Pearlin L I, Radabaugh C 1979 Age and stress: perspectives and problems. In: Fiske M (ed) Time and transitions. Jossey-Bass, San Francisco

Piaget J 1952 The origins of intelligence in children (Trans. M Cook) International University Press, New York

Reichard S, Livson F, Peterson P (1962) Aging and personality: a study of 87 older men. Wiley, New York

Reilly M 1974 Play as exploratory learning. Sage Publications, Los Angeles

Santrock J W, Bartlett H J C 1986 Developmental psychology. Brown, Iowa, W.C.

Schaie K W, Parham I A 1976 Stability of adult personality: fact or babble? Journal of Personality and Social Psychology 34: 146–158

Shaffer D R 1985 Developmental psychology. Brooks/Cole, Monterey, California

Siegler I C, George L K, Okun M A 1979 Cross-sequential analysis of adult personality. Developmental Psychology 15: 350–351

Slobin D 1971 Psycholinguistics. Scott, Foresman, Glenview, Illinois Smedslund J 1961 The acquisition of conservation of substance and weight in children: (ii) External reinforcement of conservation of weight and the operations of addition and subtraction. Scandinavian Journal of Psychology 2: 71–84

Smith G A, Brewer N 1985 Age and individual differences in correct and error reaction times. British Journal of Psychology 76: 199–203

Snow C E, Arlman-Rupp A, Hassing Y, Jobse J, Joosken J, Vorster J 1976 Mother's speech in three social classes. Journal of Psycholinguistic Research 5: 1–20

Tanner J M 1963 The regulation of human growth. Child Development 34: 817–847

Tiffany E G 1983 The developmental treatment approach. In: Hopkins H L, Smith H D (eds) Williard and Spackman's Occupational therapy, 6th edn. Lippincott, Philadelphia

Tomlinson-Keasey C, Eisert D C, Kahle L R, Hardy-Brown K, Keasy B 1979 The structure of concrete operational thought. Child Development 50: 1153–1163

Walmsley J, Margolis J 1987 Hot house people. Pan Books, London

Waterman A S, Waterman C K 1972 Relationship between ego identity status and subsequent academic behaviour: A test of the predictive validity of Marcia's categorization for identity status. Developmental Psychology 6: 179

Table 4.3

Erikson E H 1963 Childhood and society, 2nd edn. Norton, New York

Hopkins H L, Smith H D (eds) Williar and Spackman's Occupational therapy 7th edn. Lippincott, Philadelphia, section 2, p 50

Parten M B 1932 Social play among pre-school children. Journal of Abnormal Social Psychology 27: 243

Piaget J 1948 The origins of intelligence. Cook M (trans). Illinois Free Press, Glencoe

CHAPTER 5

Annett J, Kay H 1956 Skilled performance. Occupational psychology 30: 112–117

Annett J, Duncan K D, Stammers R B, Gray M J 1971 Task analysis. Training Information No 6. HMSO, London

Argyle M 1969 Social Interaction. Methuen, London

Ausubel D P 1963 The psychology of meaningful verbal learning. Grune and Stratton, New York

Bartlett F C 1943 Fatigue following highly skilled work. Proceedings of the Royal Society (B) 131: 247–257

Berne E 1966 Games people play. Andre Deutsch, London

Chomsky N 1959 Review of Skinner's verbal behavior. Language 35: 26–58

Crossman E R 1959 A theory of the acquisition of speed-skill. Ergonomics 2: 153–166

De Cecco J P 1968 The psychology of learning and instruction. Prentice-Hall, Englewood Cliffs, New Jersey

Drouet V 1983 Behaviour modification research project: occupational therapy involvement. British Journal of Occupational Therapy 46: 137–140

Fitts P M 1964 Perceptual-motor skill learning. In: Melton A W (ed) Categories of human learning. Academic Press, New York

Fitts P M, Posner M I 1967 Human performance. Brooks-Cole, Belmont, California

Fleishman E A, Hempel W E 1955 The relation between abilities and improvement with practice in a visual discrimination reaction task. Journal of Experimental Psychology 49: 301–312

Fransella F 1982 Psychology for occupational therapists. The British Psychological Society and The Macmillan Press Ltd, London

Harlow H F, Harlow M K, Meyer D R 1950 Learning motivated by a manipulation drive. Journal of Experimental Psychology 40: 228–234

Heron W T 1957 The pathology of boredom. Scientific American 196: 52–56

Hick W E 1952 On the rate of gain of information. Quarterly Journal of Experimental Psychology 4: 11–26

Hull C L 1943 Principles of behavior. Appleton-Century-Crofts, New York

James W 1890 Principles of psychology (2 vols) Macmillan, London Kelly G A 1955 The psychology of personal constructs, vols I and II Norton, New York

Kielhofner G, Burke J 1985 Components and determinants of human occupation In: Kielhofner G (ed) A model of human occupation: theory and application. Williams and Wilkins, Baltimore

Kielhofner G (ed) 1985 A model of human occupation: theory and application. William and Wilkins, Baltimore

Lovell R B 1982 Adult learning. Croom Helm, London

Maslow A H 1954 Motivation and personality. Harper & Row, New York

McClelland D C 1951 Personality. Holt, New York

Meyer A 1917 The aims and meaning of psychiatric diagnosis. American Journal of Insanity 74: 163–168

Miller J G 1960 Input overload and psychopathology. American Journal of Psychiatry 116: 695–704

Mocellin G 1984 Adaptation, coping or competence? Theoretical choices and professional decisions in occupational therapy. Proceedings of the Australian Association of Occupational Therapy, vol 2.

Naylor J C 1962 Parameters affecting the relative effectiveness of part and whole training methods: a review of the literature. US Naval Training Devices Center, New York

Oldfield R C 1959 The analysis of human skill. In: Halmos P, Iliffe A (eds) Readings in general psychology. Routledge and Kegan Paul, London

Penderry M L, Maltzman I M, West L J 1982 Controlled drinking by alcoholics? New findings and re-evaluation of a major affirmative study. Science 217: 169–175

Sackett J, Fitzgerald J 1983 An introduction to behaviour modification (Part I). British Journal of Occupational Therapy 46: 128–131

Shannon C E 1948 A mathematical theory of communication. Bell System Technical Journal 27: 379–423

Shingledecker C A 1981 Handicap and human skill. In: Holding D (ed) Human skills. Wiley, New York

Skinner B F 1938 The Behavior of organisms. Appleton-Century-Crofts, New York

Skinner B F 1957 Verbal behavior. Appleton-Century-Crofts, New York

Skinner B F 1972 Beyond freedom and dignity. Jonathan Cape, London
Snygg D, Combs A W 1949 Individual behavior. Harper and Row, New York
  (Revised edition: Combs & Snygg 1959)
Sobell M B, Sobell L C 1976 Second-year treatment outcome of alcoholics
  treated by individualised behaviour therapy: Results. Behavior Research and
  Therapy 14: 195–215
Stammers R, Patrick J 1975 The psychology of training. Methuen, London
Sutliffe P 1984 Let occupational therapy become occupational education. British
  Journal Occupational Therapy 47: 208
Wertheimer M 1945 Productive thinking. Harper, New York
White R W 1959 Motivation reconsidered: the concept of competence.
  Psychological Review 66: 297–333
White R W 1971 The urge towards competence. American Journal of
  Occupational Therapy 25(6): 271–274
Wiener N 1948 Cybernetics. Wiley, New York
Wolpe J 1958 Psychotherapy by reciprocal inhibition. Stanford University Press,
  Stanford, California
Yerxa E 1983 Audacious values: the energy source for occupational therapy
  practice. In: Kielhofner G (ed) Health through occupation. FA Davis,
  Philadelphia

CHAPTER 6

Dunton W R Jnr 1918 The principles of occupational therapy. Public Health
  Nurse 10: 320
Engelhardt H T 1974 The concepts of health and disease. In: Spicher S F (ed)
  Evaluation and explanation in the biomedical sciences. Reidell, Dordrecht
Reed K L, Sanderson S R 1980 Concepts of occupational therapy. Williams and
  Wilkins, Baltimore
Shannon P 1977 The derailment of occupational therapy. American Journal of
  Occupational Therapy 31(4): 229–234
Thompson I E 1990 Ethics In: Creek J (ed) Occupational therapy in mental
  health. Churchill Livingstone, Edinburgh
Williams G H 1984 Interpretation and compromise in coping with the experience
  of chronic illness. Unpublished Ph. D. thesis. University of Manchester
Williams G H 1986 Lay beliefs about the causes of rheumatoid arthritis: the
  implications for rehabilitation. International Rehabilitation Medicine 8: 65–68
Williams G H 1987 Disablement in the social context of daily activity.
  International Disablement Studies 9(3): 97–102
Yerxa E J 1980 Audacious values: the energy source for occupational therapy
  practice. American Journal of Occupational Therapy 14

CHAPTER 7

AOTA 1979 Representative Assembly, 59th Annual Conference (minutes)
  American Journal of Occupational Therapy 33: 781–813
Boyer J, Coleman W, Levy L, Manoly B 1989 Affective responses to activities:
  A comparative study. American Journal of Occupational Therapy 43(2): 81–88
Clark P N 1979 Human development through occupation. A philosophy and
  conceptual model for practice, Part 2. American Journal of Occupational
  Therapy 33: 577–585
Cynkin C 1979 Occupational therapy. Towards health through activities. Little,
  Brown, Boston

Cynkin C, Robinson A N 1990 Occupational therapy and activities in health. Little, Brown & Co, Boston, ch 7

Llorens L A 1981 On the meaning of activity in occupational therapy. Journal of the New Zealand Association of Occupational Therapists 21: 3–6

Llorens L A 1984 Changing balance: environment and individual. American Journal of Occupational Therapy 38: 29–34

Mosey A C 1981 Configuration of a profession. Raven Press, New York

Reed K, Sanderson S R 1980 Concepts of occupational therapy. Williams and Wilkins, Baltimore

Spahr R Paper presented to the meeting of the American Orthopsychiatric Society, March, 1965 In: Hemphill BJ (ed) 1982 The evaluation process in psychiatric occupational therapy Slack Inc, Thorofare, New Jersey

Stein J S 1979 The facets of occupational therapy: models of reward. American Journal of Occupational Therapy 23: 491–494

Turner A 1981 The practice of occupational therapy: an introduction to the treatment of physical dysfunction. Churchill Livingstone, Edinburgh

CHAPTER 8

Atchley R C 1976 The sociology of retirement. Schenkman, Cambridge, Mass

Barron F 1969 Creative person and creative process. Holt, Rinehart Winston, New York

Brown G W, Harris T 1978 Social origins of depression: a study of psychological disorder in women. Tavistock, London

Connolly J 1982 Social pretend play and social competence in preschoolers. In: Pepler E J, Rubin K (eds) The play of children: current theory and research. Karger, Basel

de Grazia S 1964 Of time, work and leisure. Twentieth Century Fund, New York

de Grazia S 1968 Environment and policy, the next fifty years. Indiana University Press, Bloomington, Indiana

Ekerdt D J, Bosse R, Levkoff S 1985 Empirical test for phases of retirement: findings from the normative ageing study. Journal of Gerontology 40: 95–101

Faughnan P 1977 The dimensions of need: a study of members of the Irish Wheelchair Association. Central Remedial Clinic, Clontarf, Dublin

Gardner G 1977 Is there a valid test of Herzberg's two-factor theory? Journal of Occupational Psychology 50: 197–204

Geist H 1968 The psychological aspects of retirement. Charles C Thomas, Springfield, Illinois

Gurney R, Taylor 1981 Research on unemployment: defects, neglect and prospects. Bulletin of the British Psychological Society 34: 349–352

Hailmann W N 1887 The education of man (abridged translation of Froebel's major work). New York

Hartley J F 1980 The impact of unemployment upon the self-esteem of managers. Journal of Occupational Psychology 53: 147–155

Havighurst R J 1982 The world of work. In: Wolman B B (ed) Handbook of developmental psychology. Prentice Hall, Englewood Cliffs, New Jersey

Herzberg F 1974 Work and the nature of man. Crosby, Lockwood, Staples, London

Hobbs Cubie S, Kaplan K L, Kielhofner G 1985 Program development. In: Kielhofner G (ed) A model of human occupation: theory and application. Williams and Wilkins, Baltimore

Hobbs Cubie S 1985 Occupational analysis. In: Kielhofner G (ed) A model of human occupation: theory and application. William and Wilkins, Baltimore

Hutt C, Bhavnani R 1976 Predictions from play. In: Bruner J S, Jolly A, Sylvia K (eds) Play. Penguin Books, New York

Kielhofner G (ed) 1985 A model of human occupation: theory and application. Williams and Wilkins, Baltimore

Lilley I M 1967 Friedrich Froebel. A selection from his writings. Cambridge University Press; Cambridge

Little C B 1976 Technical-professional unemployment: middle-class adaptability to personal crisis. Sociology Quarterly 17: 262–274

Mead M 1957 The pattern of leisure in contemporary American culture. Annals of the American Academy of Political and Social Science 313: 11–15

Meyer A 1917 The aims and meaning of psychiatric diagnosis. American Journal of Insanity 74: 163–168

Miles A 1972 The development of interpersonal relationships among long-stay patients in two hospital workshops. British Journal of Medical Psychology 45: 105–113

Montessori M 1965 Dr Montessori's own handbook (1914). Schocken, New York

Piaget J 1951 Play, dreams and imitation in childhood. Norton, New York

Nichol M 1984 Constructive activities. In: Willson M (ed) Occupational therapy in short-term psychiatry. Churchill Livingstone, Edinburgh

Parker S 1971 The future of work and leisure. Praeger, New York

Parten M 1972 Social play among preschool children. Journal of Abnormal and Social Psychology 27: 243–269

Quinn E 1980 Creativity and cognitive complexity. Social Behavior and Personality 8(2): 213–215

Ravetz C 1984 Leisure. In: Willson M (ed) Occupational therapy in short-term psychiatry. Churchill Livingstone, Edinburgh

Reichard S, Livson F, Petersen P G 1962 Ageing and personality. Wiley, New York

Reilly M 1974 Play as exploratory learning. Sage, Beverley Hills

Roberts K 1974 The changing relationship between work and leisure. In: Appleton I (ed) Leisure research and policy. Scottish Academic Press, Edinburgh

Roe A 1952 The making of a scientist. Dodd Mead, New York

Rubin K H, Fein G, Vandenberg B 1983 Play In: Hetherington EM (ed) Carmichael's manual of child psychology: social development. Wiley, New York

Shepherd G 1981 Psychological disorder and unemployment. Bulletin of the British Psychological Society 34: 345–348

Slater R 1984 Ageing. In: Gale A, Chapman A J (eds) Psychology and human problems: an introduction to applied psychology. John Wiley and Sons, Chichester

Super D 1965 The psychology of careers: an introduction to vocational development. Harper and Row, New York

Taylor F W 1947 Scientific management. Harper and Bros, New York

Wansbrough N, Cooper P 1980 Open employment after mental illness. Tavistock, London

Warnath C 1979 Vocational theories: direction to no-where. In: Weinrachs (ed) Career counselling: theoretical and practical perspectives. McGraw-Hill, New York

Whitsett D A, Winslow E K 1967 An analysis of studies critical of the motivator-hygiene theory. Personnel Psychology 20: 4

Wing J K, Brown G W 1970 Institutionalism and schizophrenia: a comparative study of three mental hospitals 1960–1968. Cambridge University Press, Cambridge

CHAPTER 9

Audit Commission Report 1986 Making a reality of community care. HMSO, London

Barton R 1966 Institutional neurosis, 2nd edn John Wright and Sons, Bristol

Black J 1982 Mental hospitals. In: Brearley P (ed) Leaving residential care. Tavistock, London

Blom-Cooper L 1989 Occupational therapy: an emerging profession in health care (Report of a Commission of Inquiry) Duckworth, London

Bowlby J 1953 Child care and the growth of love. Pelican Books, London

Brearley P (ed) 1982 Leaving residential care. Tavistock, London

Central Statistical Office 1981 Social trends, no. 11. HMSO, London

Clarke B 1990 Cerebral palsy in Ireland. Slanuacht: the Journal of the National Rehabilitation Board, May: 14

Clough R 1981 Old age homes. Allen and Unwin, London

Clough R 1982 Residential work. MacMillan Press, London

Cooper D 1967 Psychiatry and anti-psychiatry. Tavistock, London

Curtis Committee Report 1946 Report of the care of children committee. HMSO, London

Department of Health and Social Security 1975 Better services for the mentally ill (White Paper). HMSO, London

Department of Health and Social Security 1988 Community care: agenda for action, (The Griffiths Report). HMSO, London

Department of Health and Social Security 1989 Caring for people: community care in the next decade and beyond. HMSO, London

Deutsch A 1948 Shame of the States. Harcourt and Brace, New York

DHSS 1981a Care in action. A handbook of policies and priorities for the health and personal social services in England. HMSO, London

Goffman E 1961 Asylums: essays on the social situation of mental patients and other inmates. Anchor Books, Doubleday, New York

Goldie N 1977 The division of labour among the mental health professions – a negotiated or imposed order? In: Stacey M (ed) Health and the division of labour. Croom Helm, London

House of Commons Social Services Committee on 'Community Care with special reference to adult mentally ill and mentally handicapped people'. HC 13: 1984–85

Jordan B 1976 Freedom and the welfare state. Routledge and Kegan Paul, London

Lapping A 1974 Community action. Fabian Society, London

Mooney R 1982 Guide for the disabled. Paperfacts, Ward River Press, Swords, Co. Dublin

Wallace M 1988 Did Edward have to die? Sunday Times Magazine, July 24th

Subject index

Author index